This is a work of fiction. Names, characters, places, and incidents are either the product of the author's imagination and are used fictitiously. Any resemblance to actual persons, living or dead is coincidental.

The Magician's Legacy
Peter Sharp Legal Adventure #7

Magic Lamp

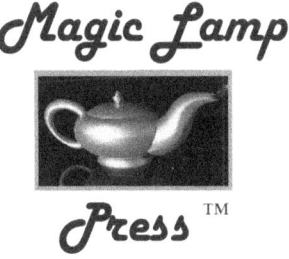

Press ™

ISBN: 1-882629-15-9

The Complete Peter Sharp Legal Mystery Series

Single Jeopardy

...By Reason of Sanity

A Class Action

Conspiracy of Innocence

...Until Proven Innocent

The Common Law

The Magician's Legacy

The Reluctant Jurist

The Final Case

An Element of Peril

A Good Alibi

Legally Dead

I0546466

FOREWORD

If this is the first Peter Sharp Legal Mystery that you're reading, it might help you to know a little background information about the characters.

Peter Sharp's wife threw him out of their home (which she actually owned), due to a conflict of their philosophies about legal representation: Peter being a defender of those poor, unfortunate people 'wrongfully' accused of crimes, and his wife Myra a prosecutor with the District Attorney's office.

Peter ultimately wound up living on a dilapidated old boat in Marina del Rey, and when his former classmate/employer Melvin Braunstein died in a plane crash, Peter inherited a failing law practice, an office manager (Melvin's twelve-year old step-daughter Suzi, a Chinese computer genius) and her huge St. Bernard. Peter was appointed legal guardian, and through a series of misfortunes that miraculously

3

worked out, wound up living with Suzi and her dog on a beautiful 50-foot Grand Banks trawler-yacht.

When Peter isn't swilling Patrón Margaritas at one of the marina's local watering holes, he's usually involved in some losing legal case that little Suzi will inevitably solve, leaving Peter with the impression that he's really as good as he thinks he is.

Along the way in each legal adventure, Peter usually winds up butting heads with his ex-wife, who Suzi adores and is constantly scheming to get back into the Sharp household. There's also Stuart Schwartzman, Peter's old friend and frequent client, who is the most entrepreneurial person in Southern California – and Jack Bibberman, the best private investigator Peter ever met.

All of the Peter Sharp Legal Mysteries are summarized at the end of this book, and if you're curious about them, more details (plus photos) are at
http://www.petersharpbooks.com

Magic Lamp Press
Venice, California

INTRODUCTION

The sinking of the Titanic in 1912 affected me, because even though I hadn't been born yet, I lost a good friend... someone I respected, admired, and wanted to be just like in some ways.

His name was Jacques Futrelle, and at the age of 37, he was travelling with his wife in the Titanic's first-class cabin number C-123.

When the boat sank, Mr. Futrelle managed to get his wife into one of the lifeboats, so she survived. He didn't.

Other than the fact that he was a human being and didn't deserve the fate that befell him, he was also a talented author, and wrote the story that influenced my life from the day that I first read it: one of the most famous locked-room mysteries of all time, **The Problem in Cell 13.**

If you're a fan of locked-room mysteries, then I strongly suggest that you read Futrelle's Cell 13 story as well as John

5

Dickson Carr's **The Hollow Man**, which was the main inspiration for the present Peter Sharp Legal Mystery in this book.

The above-mentioned stories of Futrelle and Carr, along with E.A. Poe's **the Gold Bug** and all the Sherlock Holmes, Nero Wolfe and other detectives, got me hooked on mysteries - and to my delight there is no known cure for this addiction.

All of the locked-room mysteries I've encountered have involved a victim who either died in a room that was allegedly inaccessible, unescapable from, or with a misinterpreted timeline. That's why I decided to eliminate all the excuses: in this story, the crime was actually witnessed by observers... and then the murderer disappeared into thin air, before their eyes.

Got you hooked? Good! Start reading now, and see if you can figure out the solution to this baffling locked-room Peter Sharp Legal mystery before little Suzi does.

Gene Grossman

THE MAGICIAN'S LEGACY

1

Several years ago a network television station aired some shows that featured a masked magician who dared to reveal secrets about how the most popular magic tricks and illusions are performed. He wore the mask as protection from alleged physical threats from fellow magicians who felt betrayed. I watched part of the first show, but skipped the rest of it and its several sequels because I just don't want to know how it's done.

I love magic. Every time I watch a magician perform I turn into a little kid, with my mouth and eyes wide open. I enjoy being fooled, and the more I'm tricked, the more I like it. Knowing how it's done would spoil the fun for me, and I don't want that to happen.

It looks like not everyone is like me. They're nosy. They want to know how the magicians do it. People like that suffer from a personality disorder that prevents them from believing someone is smarter than they are. They refuse to accept the fact that they can be fooled by another mere mortal... they selfishly push to find out what the 'trick' that confused them was, so they can then regain their fragile confidence and once again believe that they are superior beings, only having been temporarily fooled by some unfair gimmick that they now know about.

And as for the people who do the tricks, whenever I encounter some guy with the adjective 'great' preceding his name, one that invariably ends in a vowel, I want to be entertained. I want to be fooled. I want to see that rabbit come out of a hat, the colored silks, the self-repairing rope and the three rings that come apart and go back together again. I love it. And of course at my age, it's even better if the magician has some long-legged female assistant in high heels that helps in the misdirection. It certainly works every time with me, but I'm a normal forty-three-year-old male lawyer. It doesn't work for Suzi, the little Chinese cupie doll I live with.

She's a computer genius and the brains behind our law firm... the one that was started by her stepfather and is now headed up by me, due to a fatal airplane accident that not only left me in charge of the law practice, but also as her legal guardian. We both live aboard a 50-foot Grand Banks trawler yacht here in Marina del Rey California, along with Suzi's huge Saint Bernard that I call Bernie, because he's got some Chinese name that I can't pronounce.

The kid doesn't have many friends her age, but she does see another little girl named Lotus Chang, whose mother Michelle is a customer at Murray's Chinese restaurant, around the corner on Washington Boulevard, where Suzi's mother Jasmine was the manager. Jasmine was having trouble with her citizenship status, so a customer at the restaurant, and old law school classmate of mine named Melvin Braunstein, helped out by marrying her. When Jasmine was killed in an automobile accident about a year later, Melvin did the legal work for his stepdaughter and succeeded in settling it for quite a bit. As a result, Suzi is the richest little girl in the Marina.

When Melvin perished in a private plane crash, his Will appointed me as Suzi's legal guardian. A year later, I succeeded in getting a huge settlement for her from the distributor of faulty counterfeit airplane parts: that enriched the kid's trust fund by another couple of million dollars. As official administrator of her bank accounts I get paid a whopping CEO salary of one dollar per year, and our little law practice seems to be thriving, so we're living on a beautiful yacht named the 'Suzi B' that I don't even know how to start the engine of. The fees keep coming in, I have my big Yellow Hummer to ride around in, and there's an alcoholic broad named Laverne living on a houseboat near us who is an altogether different kind of hummer that I ride occasionally. Life is good.

Michelle Chang invited Suzi to Lotus's surprise 11th birthday party, so I'm all alone on the boat tonight trying to get some research done, with a 200-pound Saint Bernard asleep across my feet. Unfortunately, I wasn't invited to the party, which is too bad, because I understand that Mrs. Chang hired a professional magician from the Magic Castle to come and entertain the kids. I tried to tell her that whenever a magician is around, I'm a kid too, but it didn't work.

When the kid's here, we often have some gourmet Chinese dinners delivered from Murray's, by a group of four young fellows nicknamed the 'Asian Boys' who work evenings at the restaurant, and varnish boats during the day. With no kid and no Asian Boys, my dinner tonight will consist of the usual pot of gruel that I've perfected over the years. The recipe involves eight ounces of elbow macaroni plus the addition of one or more of several flavoring items that can vary between non-fat cottage cheese, non-fat baked beans, non-fat butter, green peas, low-fat cream of mushroom soup, non-fat vegetarian chili, or whatever else I happen to find within reaching distance.

Whatever the final mixture is, it all gets topped off with a generous sprinkling of imitation Parmesan cheese and some garlic salt, and most of it never makes it to the table because it gets eaten right near the stove. I've been told that single men are the only variety of humans that are known to eat standing up.

This time there's enough 'Pasta ala Peter' prepared to be finished up sitting down in the yacht's main saloon. Like so many other uninformed boaters, I used to call it the 'salon,' but some balding old jerk with a fifty-foot sailboat on our dock bawled me out when he heard me call it that, and demanded that I use its correct designation. I try to show respect to my know-it-all elder, so now it's the main 'saloon.'

The dog is always alert whenever I'm eating, because he's on constant 'crumb

11

patrol,' but I don't mind him around on evenings like this because he's an excellent listener. Tonight's seminar is on the double job that's usually required whenever a lawyer takes on certain types of cases, one of them being for legal malpractice. The extra work is because not only does the new lawyer have to prove that the original lawyer was guilty of screwing up, but he must also show that if the case was handled properly that the client could have actually won. This means that not only do you have to destroy the first lawyer, but you also have to go ahead and almost completely re-create the first trial, showing how it should have been won. And that's the reason I don't take cases like that.

Both the dinner and the dissertation have been completed and not one living thing in the room disagrees with me about either... another successful dinner lecture.

The birthday party must be over now because Mrs. Chang just called to let me know that she'll be bringing Suzi back to the Marina. I was supposed to pick her up, but I like to think that this favor is motivated by a combination of her wanting to give Lotus more time with Suzi - and her desire to see me. Ego self-inflation has always been one of my strong suits.

When they all arrive at the boat and dump some party stuff on table I see that once again my thoughts were wrong, because it's Mrs. Chang who's the one spending more time with Suzi. Michelle is in the IRS's Intelligence and Enforcement Division, and is fascinated by all the crime-fighting software that the kid has 'collected' on her computer, as a result of being so closely associated with my ex-wife (who is now the elected District Attorney of Los Angeles County) and all the cops who consider her a mascot. This mascot status is because of the kid's daily noon appearances at the Murray's Chinese restaurant around the corner, where her mother used to work. It's also the place where squad cars from all the local police agencies converge for lunch, or as Suzi informs me, a 'Code 7,' which in police-speak means 'out of service, to eat.'

One remarkable feature about this Chinese restaurant is an official-looking sign posted in the men's room that I've been told commands 'employees to their wash hands before returning to work.' Good idea, but in a Chinese restaurant with Chinese immigrant employees, you'd think they might have the sign in some language other than Spanish.

Word about Suzi's computer skills and searching abilities have gotten around and enabled our firm to pick up quite a few clients and gather some future favors from local law enforcement groups. Her popularity is also due to some of the missing forms from our file cabinet that were probably used to help many of those cops defend the divorce actions that police wives are wont to file.

Unlike Suzi, little Lotus Chang is quite talkative around me, so while her mother is busy with my boatmate in the foreward stateroom, I get a full narrative about how the birthday party went. Listening to this little girl rattle on and on makes me more appreciative of the fact that Suzi rarely talks to me, opting instead to make most communications by 'dog-mail,' which consists of tucking a message into the Saint Bernard's collar and sending him to me.

Most of Lotus' story is about the other kids that attended the party. Not interested. She goes on to provide me with a detailed list of every present she received at the party, complete with a full description of each and every gift-giver. Still not interested. My eyelids are now getting heavy.

Among the party debris still defacing our beautiful expensive teak table are some Polaroid photos taken at the party, and one of them I find particularly interesting because it shows a strikingly attractive woman standing next to an older man. At first I thought that they must be the mother and grandfather of one of the kids attending the party, but as Lotus drones on, she informs me that the photo in my hand is Mister Robert Balscomb, previous owner of the Changs' house.

Lotus says that Balscomb stopped by with Marian, his housekeeper. The reason for their invitation to the party was that Marian is Michelle Chang's former porcelain-painting teacher, and the person who originally told Mrs. Chang about Balscomb's house being for sale. Michelle wanted to show off how her porcelain collection is displayed, so Mister Balscomb came along to do the driving and give Mrs. Chang some pointers on features of the 'safe room' where she keeps her collection. When Balscomb owned the house he paid big bucks to convert the den into what security experts call a 'panic room,' complete with bulletproof walls and emergency communication devices. He's obviously either paranoid, or has a very checkered past he's afraid might catch up with him.

Lotus notices that I can't seem to stop looking at the picture of Balscomb and his companion, and surprises me.

"Gee, that's funny... Marian kept looking at your picture too."

"What are you talking about Lotus?

"That picture of you and Suzi. You know, the one you guys took at her birthday party last year. She gave it to me for my 'friends' collection, and when Marian, the lady in the picture with Mister Balscomb, saw it, she kept looking at it the same way you're looking at that picture of her."

This is interesting. It's almost like computer dating, because we seem to be interested in each other's pictures. Maybe I should call her. This might present a slight problem. Somewhere in the back of my mind I get the feeling that Lotus' mother Michelle might be interested in me. That's flattering, but I could never get involved with anyone connected with the IRS... but at the same time, I don't want to hurt her feelings. I'm going to see this Marian, but it will have to be a covert operation at first.

Lotus says that Suzi didn't think much of Mister Robert Balscomb. If you're not a uniformed law enforcement officer it's tough to get her respect. She's a cop groupie, so it's not surprising to hear she didn't warm up to Balscomb. What does surprise me is hearing that Balscomb was so impressed by the magician entertaining the kids that he stayed for the whole performance and seemed to enjoy it as much as the kids did. He also made sure to get one of the magician's business cards before leaving.

The Changs are leaving the boat now and my phone is ringing. It's my close friend Stuart, who rarely calls just to say hello. He's the most entrepreneurial person I know, and now has at least five successful businesses going that I'm aware of. Whenever I see his familiar telephone number on my caller I.D. display I assume it's either because he needs some emergency legal advice or wants to tell me all about some new business he's going to start up.

"Hello Stuart, what's up?"

"Peter, I'm angry."

"Okay Stu, why don't you just calm down and tell me about it."

"You're going to think it's too trivial and you'll probably laugh at me."

"Stuart, I promise I won't laugh. I've been practicing law and listening to clients for almost twenty years now, and my legal bedside manner has developed to the point where I can control any urge to laugh at what I'm being told, so go ahead, let's hear about it. Does it have anything to do with money?"

"Yes Pete, it does."

"All right, now we're getting to the heart of the matter. What's the amount?"

There's silence on the line as Stuart hesitates with his answer. This probably means that the amount he got screwed out of is so large that he's embarrassed to tell me. "C'mon Stu. You called me, so if you won't tell me the amount, then I'd like to get off the phone and go back to some things I'm doing around the boat."

"Seventy cents."

Stuart never fails to surprise me. "Stuart, I know in my heart that the amount can't be bothering you, because next to Suzi you're one of the richest people I know. There's must be something else that's bothering you about that trifling sum, so please, let me know what it is."

"You're right Pete. It's not the amount, it's the principle of the thing. I picked up a chopped salad to-go at a restaurant. It was eight dollars and fifty cents."

"So?"

"So, they charged me sales tax on it!"

"What's the big deal? You pay sales tax on everything else you buy that's not for resale, so why complain this time?"

"Peter, you went to law school. Didn't they teach you that there's not supposed to be sales tax charged on food to-go?"

"Sorry Stu, I must have been absent that day. Are you sure about the law on that matter?"

"Not exactly, but I pick up a lot of carry-out food, and to the best of my recollection, this is the first time I've ever been charged sales tax on it. I should think that while the exact percentage amount might vary between jurisdictions, the main policy decision of whether or not it's due on food-to-go is a statewide decision and should be consistent."

"So what do you intend to do about it? Turn them in to the State Board of Equalization, or Franchise Tax Board, or whatever agency handles that stuff? Or are you planning some huge class action on behalf of all the taxpayers in the State? Either way, I don't think I'm with you on this one. At least not with the facts the way they are to this point."

"Oh yeah? Well what would you do if you were me?"

"First, I'd go back to that restaurant and show them two receipts: one from another nearby restaurant that didn't charge the tax on a similar item to-go, and also the receipt from their own register on which the tax was added. I'd also make sure that I talked to someone in the restaurant who was in charge, because there's always the possibility that the sale was rung up by a new employee or someone else there who just made a common mistake and pressed a wrong classification button on the cash register.

"If you handle it like a gentleman, I'm sure you'll get a happy conclusion. If a mistake was actually made, any competent manager should probably apologize to you and might even offer you a dinner on the house for pointing it out to them. But first and most important, please go to the State's local tax office and find out what the law really is. It's obvious that one of those restaurants made a mistake, and it's either the one that charged you, or the one that didn't. I think you owe it to them as a neighbor to point out the error to the wrongdoer, and not just rush to turn them in or file a lawsuit."

Stuart grudgingly agrees with me and says he'll check out the law. After hanging up I start going through several party favors spread around on the table, hoping there's some leftover birthday cake included, and happen upon a business card that announces 'The Great Schwartzi." This is obviously the party magician's card. The surprising part is what's written on the blank back side of the card. It's a local address, with a scribbled note that says 'Suzi, I'll expect you at my house tomorrow at one P.M.'

2

I've been thinking about it all night and this is not something I tend to approve of. Who is this Great Schwartzi, and why is Suzi going to his house? Without knowing more about this guy I have no intention of letting the kid go over there alone, and I'm not interested in being the chaperone. This calls for an afternoon meeting, so I prepare a note, go into the kitchen area of the boat – the area that I've been instructed to call 'the galley' by that old know-it-all down the dock, and shake a box of dog biscuits.

The noise generated by his snack food rattling in the box brings the dog out before the third shake. Now that I have his attention, I slip the message under his collar and a biscuit in his mouth. Not having any more use for me, he returns to the forward stateroom - the little princess' private domain.

Uncharacteristically, the kid decides to actually come out and address me in person. The rare times this happens I'm usually in for a lecture, and this time is no different.

"I appreciate your concern, but I do know about this man. His real name is Sheldon Schwartz and he mentioned that his birthday is on October 9th. If you remember, Dr. Sheldon Eidoch, one of the students you had in that Bar review course you were teaching, mentioned to me that the name 'Sheldon' was very popular with Jewish families during the period between 1935 and 1945, so I checked birth dates during that decade and now know that the Great Schwartzi aka Sheldon Schwartz was born in 1941 in Kansas City, and was fingerprinted in California in 1971 when he applied for his license as a real estate salesman. He has no criminal record and donates a lot of his time entertaining kids at the Los Angeles Children's Hospital.

"The reason I am going to his house is to start my magic education and to talk about a possible business arrangement with him."

"You're going to be a professional magician? What happened to Harvard Law School and hiring me and Myra as associates in your law firm?"

This provokes her predictable eye-roll, indicating that I just don't get it.

"No, silly. You and Myra will still have jobs waiting for you... I want to learn about magic because it's the art of mis-direction, and that's what happens when clues to solving a crime are hard to find. You're being mis-directed by red herrings and lying suspects. I want to learn how to cut through all of that."

"Okay, so you won't be a professional magician. That's the public's loss. What's the deal with a business arrangement? Is this something you're doing on your own, or will you be involving our law firm in it?"

"I'm not at liberty to discuss the details at this time, but rest assured that the law firm will not be involved or affected at all."

That having been said, she does an about-face and leads her beast back to the foreward stateroom. As she walks away, she tosses one of her throwaway lines at me.

"And don't prepare any of that pasta mess tonight. We'll be eating normal food at six P.M."

That's the best news I've heard all week. The Asian Boys will probably be here by five thirty to set the table and put the food in the oven for re-heating. As for her business deal with the Great Schwartzi, I'm the trustee of her accounts, and the court requires that anything she wants to spend a significant amount of money on must be approved by me, so I guess I'll find out the details soon enough.

Once she and the dog have left the boat for their first magic lesson, I call my ex-wife Myra. It's been a while since she downsized the household by exiling me to an old cabin cruiser in our back yard, but I don't hold it against her. As a result of that forced move, I renewed my acquaintance with Melvin Braunstein and ultimately wound up living here in the Marina.

I used some devious strategy to convince her opponent to drop out of the race, so Myra had no difficulty in getting elected to the office of District Attorney, and we both now live in a state of mutual co-existence, while Suzi continues her perpetual transparent efforts to get Myra and I back together again. The two of them talk on the telephone at least once or twice a day, and I get the feeling that like the dog, I'm just another 190-pound male animal that happens to be around.

Suzi has Myra's private office number, and I'm using it.

"Hello Peter."

"How did you know it was me?"

"Because Suzi's number appeared on my caller ID display, and she never calls at this time of day. What do you want, other than sex, which is no longer an option for you?"

"Don't flatter yourself. I never sleep with prosecutors. I need you to check someone out. His name is the Great Schwartzi."

"All right, this conversation is now over. I've had enough of your humor to last me a lifetime Petey, and I have work to do."

I really don't like it when she calls me that, but if that's what I have to put up with to talk to her, then it's worth it. "Whoa kid, hold on. The Great Schwartzi is the stage name used by a guy named Sheldon Schwartz. He's a magician that the kid met at a birthday party yesterday and she's gone to his house this afternoon."

"You let her go there alone?"

"No. She took the dog with her. It's only a mile or so away so they drove over there in her electric cart. She says she ran him through, but I'd like you to have your office do a more thorough background check on this guy."

"What's going on? Why is she going over to this guy's house? Is he a client or something?"

"Not exactly. She wants to learn about magic."

"Magic? Magic? What are you talking about? I thought she was going to be a Harvard lawyer and hire the both of us. I don't know about you, but I do not intend to wear a Playboy bunny costume with fish-net hose and high heels, to be a magician's assistant."

"Not to worry, our futures as lawyers are secure... but if you ever change your mind about that outfit, please call me."

There's a brief silence while I listen to the now familiar sound of her fuming. This means that I may be talking to a dial tone soon. "She thinks that knowledge of magic will help her crime-solving skills so I'll let her go through with it until she starts wearing a cape." Success. She's still on the line, so I give her whatever details I have about the great Jewish magician. Come to think of it, maybe he's really in the right profession. If memory serves me correctly the greatest of them all was Harry Houdini, and he was also Jewish, having been born in Budapest Hungary as Ehrich Weiss. I'm pretty sure he was Jewish because his father was a rabbi there. Now that my apprehensions about Sheldon Schwartz have been slightly relieved, my curiosity returns to this Balscomb fellow, why he took the magician's card and why he needs a safe room.

Hmmmn. Maybe this could be an opportunity to kill two birds with one stone. I could get to know Balscomb's housekeeper Marian, and during a casual conversation find out why her boss is so security conscious. One thing I've learned from trying cases in court is that you never ask a question you don't know the answer to, so I'd better do some homework first and learn something about those types of secure rooms.

Some time ago I made the acquaintance of Victor Gutierrez, who has become both a friend and a valuable associate. He operates a private autopsy business in the San Gabriel Valley, and the firm's name is also his telephone number: 1800AUTOPSY.

I was taken aback at first by the thought of a person who specializes in driving around picking up bodies and doing post mortems in his office. It reminds me of a doctor Frankenstein-type of profession, but after talking to him I learned that what he does provides a valuable service requested by many families and insurance companies. The County Coroner's office usually only performs autopsies when there might be a crime involved. They're not interested in medical malpractice, disguised suicides or other types of death that can lead to serious civil actions. Victor and his staff are experienced forensic scientists and our firm has used their services once or twice in the past, mostly as an independent CSI unit for criminal defense matters.

I imagine that if anyone knows about 'safe-rooms' it's Victor, because if a question concerns security or forensic investigation, he's my go-to guy. I hope he doesn't think me rude for continuously refusing invitations to come and see his facility. That's why the standard definition of a 'lawyer' is 'someone who can't stand the sight of blood.'

After a lengthy telephone conversation Victor succeeds in providing me with a college education in 'safe rooms' and I now realize how important they might be to heads of state or other tremendously important people, but still don't know why Robert Balscomb needs one.

It's understandable if an A-list celebrity or high-ranking politician prefers to have some protection, or a multi-millionaire wants safety from burglars, but to the best of my knowledge, Balscomb is neither of these. All of my Internet searching has failed to turn up anything about him. This is a job for Jack Bibberman, a guy who saved my rear-end a while back by testifying truthfully at a State Bar hearing, and since then has been a trusted friend and private investigator for our law firm. It's probably none of my business, but this safe-room stuff has peaked my curiosity, so I might as well spend a few bucks and further my general education.

I call Jack, give him Balscomb's present and past addresses, and tell him to spend some time finding out about the guy and what he might be afraid of. And for purely personal reasons, I also ask him to get me the Balscomb residence's unlisted telephone number.

That's enough work for today. Now I'm going to catch up on some reading and get in the mood for a gourmet Chinese meal. The Marina rents out some houseboats, and one of them on our dock is occupied by a woman named Laverne, who I've become quite familiar with. It's hard to guess what her age is, because she's been self-embalming herself for the past decade or so, and that has kept her quite well preserved. Even though, I'd say that she'll never see thirty-five again, and may have even hit the big four-o. Nevertheless, she's very nice to me, and after dinner tonight I'll be walking over to the Marina del Rey Liquor Store to pick up a box of Laverne's favorite wine, and then enjoy the evening on her houseboat. I justify this dalliance because Myra won't have anything to do with me, I'm afraid of Michelle's IRS, and Marian is still waiting in the wings.

Another reason I enjoy Laverne's houseboat is because it's like going to another country... some exotic place like Morocco, or one of those foreign places you only read about or see in an old black-and-white noir movie. This is due to Laverne's unique 'early gaudy' style of decorating. She had the uncanny ability to have turned her saloon, and I use the word figuratively, into an exact replica of an ancient third-world whore-house, complete with fringed tiffany lamps, red velvet flocked wallpaper, beaded doorway curtains, burning incense, and satin sheets. The only thing that brings you back to good old U. S. of A. is her television set, which is usually tuned in to one of her favorite reality shows. There's nothing like a crappy TV reality show to remind you what country you're in, our land of the free and home of the knave.

3

I don't know what Laverne does for a living, but she must do something, because early every morning she gets picked up before eight by the same husky guy who also brings her back to the Marina at dinnertime. Having seen the way she embalms herself with cheap wine, I would guess she lost her driver's license because of some drunk driving convictions and convinced that guy she probably works with to carpool each day.

Somewhere in the back of my mind I seem to remember having a nice evening, but it's still all a blur. As usual, Laverne left a few slices of greasy French toast out on the table for me, and I'm now trying to get one of them down. The houseboat is rocking slightly but I don't see anyone outside the window or hear anyone walking on the boat.

As the door gets pushed open I look down and see that a dog-mail is being delivered. Not having received a telephone call from me asking to get bailed out of jail, both the kid and her dog know that if I'm not on board for the night, that I'm usually 'visiting' Laverne. I remove a message from the maildog's collar and he immediately leaves the boat. Ordinarily he would wait for a tip that takes the form of some morsel for him to eat, but the last time he made a morning delivery to me on Laverne's boat I tossed him a slice of her French toast and he hasn't waited around for a tip since then.

I blot some grease off of my fingers and open the folded paper. It's a copy of Jack Bibberman's email that's a preliminary report on his findings about Robert Balscomb. From what Jack has learned, Balscomb is unmarried and lives with Michelle Chang's friend Marian, who has been his housekeeper for over twenty years now. The only other person living there is Balscomb's nephew Jessie, a twenty-year-old young man who occasionally attends classes at Santa Monica Junior College. They all occupy the large three-story home that Balscomb had custom built in Marina del Rey's exclusive *Peninsula* area, just off the sand and overlooking the Grand Canal and Pacific Ocean.

Jack also mentions that he's now in the process of getting plans of the house from the Department of Building & Safety, so that we can see what he built in the way of a safe room. He says he'll report to me again when the complete background check he requested comes back.

At the bottom of the e-mail copy is a hand-written note:

Peter:
If this has nothing to do with an open case, then please have Jack bill you personally.
The office manager

Nothing gets past that little pre-teen snoop.

Myra finished her investigation of the Great Schwartzi and it looks like he's just a harmless guy in his late sixties who performs magic. The report says that at one time he was quite famous and made a bundle inventing illusions that he would sell for big bucks to other famous magicians. Many of the books he's written over the years on the art of magic are still being sold on Amazon.com and Abebooks.com, so in addition to party performances and giving lessons, he's also got some royalties coming in.

- - - - - - -

Suzi has been studying with him for two months now, but the only magic performances she gives are for her friend Lotus and the dog. I haven't received any requests from the bank for a withdrawal from her accounts, so I guess that if she's investing any money with the magician, it must be coming from some regular account where she stashes her fees for investigation and all the other stuff she does on the side for God only knows who.

Jack Bibberman completed his background check of Robert Balscomb and impressed me with a thorough history of his family that goes back almost a hundred years. Balscomb's father R. Balscomb Sr. was born in 1910, and in 1928 started working for the Hathaway Manufacturing Company, a cotton mill.

In the 1950's, Balscomb Sr.'s boss decided to merge his company with another cotton mill, called Berkshire Fine Spinning Associates. Under the terms of the merger, investors received 4 shares of stock in the new company for each share of Hathaway stock they exchanged.

Because Balscomb Sr. had accumulated 300 shares during his twenty-plus years of employment, he received 1200 shares of the new company, which was growing in size and business capacity on a regular basis.

About ten years later in 1962, a bright young investor named Warren Buffet noticed how well the cotton mill's business was doing. He thought it was undervalued at only $15 a share, so he started buying into the company, and in a short period of time the stock went up from $15 to $18 a share.

A former executive of the company had a slight problem with drinking and gambling and asked Balscomb Sr. to lend him a thousand dollars. As collateral for the loan, he offered to let Balscomb hold his 700 shares of stock, then worth over twelve thousand dollars. As expected with a drunken gambler, the loan was never repaid and after numerous extensions and pleading, Balscomb Sr. had no other choice than to consider the collateral forfeited and had the shares transferred to his own name, bringing his holdings up to a full one thousand shares.

Being an honorable man, Balscomb borrowed money against the shares and sent a check to the drunk's family for ten thousand dollars. The debtor took the money and promptly deserted his family.

As they say, the rest is history. Anyone familiar with the stock market knows that Berkshire Hathaway is now the most expensive stock in the world, sometimes trading for as much as ninety thousand dollars a share. The stock and dividends that Robert Balscomb inherited from his father is now worth close to one hundred million dollars, and sits in various trust accounts and other investments that pay Robert Balscomb a very comfortable income of approximately a half million dollars each month. Now it's easy to see why money was no object when he had his house built with that safe-room installed. It must have cost him almost two months' allowance.

Jack dug further into the court records and learned that on several occasions Balscomb obtained restraining orders against some angry people who claimed that Balscomb stole their family's money. They were probably descendants of the drunken debtor who felt entitled to the benefit of his stock investment.

With Jack's report now complete, it's easy to see why Robert Balscomb wanted to be safe in his own home.

Balscomb must also really be interested in magic because Jack says that on at least three occasions he saw the

Great Schwartzi arrive in a cab and go into Balscomb's house, and that he would usually stay in there for at least two hours. It looks like magic lessons seem to be the latest fad. Jack used his 10 mega-pixel digital camera to get Schwartzi's picture, and he emailed it to me. This magician is one strange looking guy, with a big bushy head of hair, full beard, and dressed in all black, complete with a cape. Not a bad outfit for the stage, or in Transylvania, but a little out of fashion for walking around in Marina del Rey.

Our personal line rings. It's a number my caller ID doesn't recognize. Suzi must be busy with the dog, so I answer it and get a pleasant surprise.

"Hello Mister Sharp. We've never met, but I'm Marian, a friend of Michelle Chang. I met your Suzi at Lotus' birthday party recently and was calling to check with her to find out if she minds making her appointment with the Great Schwartzi tomorrow. He'll also be giving lessons to my employer, Mister Robert Balscomb."

"Oh yeah, I saw a picture of the two of you taken at the party. Lotus showed it to me. I understand you've also seen a picture of me. Say, I've got a crazy idea. Now that we've seen each other and know that we're almost neighbors, why don't we get together for a cup of coffee some afternoon?

"We've got something in common: we're both on the outside looking in on people who are crazy about magic. Maybe we can compare notes."

It worked. We agree to meet at the Cheesecake Factory next week while the students are having a magic lesson. We also decide to be very discreet about it. I'm looking forward to this... being with an attractive woman who can cook, sew and keep a house clean. If she's lucky, I may give her some of my special pasta recipes.

On a recent visit to the boat by Michelle Chang and her daughter Lotus, the young one started bending my ear with some gossip. She overheard Marian telling her mother about how Schwartzi was fascinated by the security of Balscomb's safe room and how he thought he could design a plan to get in and out of it. From what Lotus says, the housekeeper told Michelle that Balscomb had a good laugh when he heard that plan and offered to make a side bet with Schwartzi any time he might like to give his plan a try.

As a devout fan of the locked-room mystery genre, I understand Schwartzi's fascination with the concept of a safe-room. Most locked-room mysteries involve just that: a locked room. There's no particular requirement that it be a bulletproof, soundproof, steel-doored, theft-proof place. Any plain old room with a locked door and no apparent way for anyone to enter, commit the crime, and exit afterwards will usually suffice.

The only thing that comes close to what Schwartzi probably has in mind is the famous Jacques Futrelle short story *The Problem of Cell 13*, where Professor S.F.X. Van Dusen, the 'thinking machine,' promises to get himself out of the infamous escape-proof Chisholm prison's death-cell. I guess that Schwartzi couldn't find a prison to cooperate with him, so he opted for the secure room in Balscomb's house. I'll be very interested to see what type of illusion he comes up with if he ever pulls it off. This will be another thing for me to discuss with Marian when we have coffee.

The Cheesecake Factory is a very popular chain of restaurants here in California, and whenever they open a new one it's usually packed from the first day and stays that way forever. Fortunately, we have one across the street from where our boat is tied up, so it's a short walk for me to go and meet with Marian.

We have a very enjoyable lunch and an interesting conversation, but she seems reluctant to talk about Balscomb. The only details I can get out of her without using a thumb-screw are that her mother started working for the Balscomb family when she was a small child, and after her mother died from some illness, Marian stayed to carry on the tradition of service to the Balscomb household.

Okay, I can live with the lack of information from her. At least she agreed to meet with me on her next night off. This will be another interesting situation, because if our relationship gets to the next level, we'll have to figure out some place to spend time together. Good thing the Foghorn Motel is next door to the Cheesecake Factory and Marina del Rey Liquor Store.

When we're through eating I order a few pieces of cheesecake to go. I know that the kid loves sweets, and I won't mind having a nice dessert for breakfast tomorrow morning. The waitress brings me a bag with the sweets in it and I tell her to add the extra amount to my credit card. I also make a concerted effort to not inspect the bill to see if she added sales tax to the cheesecake to-go. The other part of my dessert is a good-bye kiss from Marian as she gets into her car.

I took some time out to surf the internet and came up with some interesting info for my friend Stuart. Searching through California's Revenue and Taxation Code, I learned that section 6359 contains a list of all the foods that are taxable, and the exemptions that apply.

If Stuart picked up only a chopped salad, then he shouldn't have had to pay sales tax on his carry-out order unless the restaurant provides parking spaces and outdoor tables for people to eat their to-go orders.

I don't know what restaurant he was referring to, but as long as the carry-out item isn't what the Board of Equalization classifies as a 'hot prepared food product,' meaning anything that's meant to be served at a temperature that is higher than the room temperature of the room where it is sold, then it should be a sales tax exempt carry-out.

This particular code section is one of the most complicated ones I've ever read because it classifies foods of so many types and bases the reasons for taxation on so many variables. I think that as long as

Stuart sticks to only a cold salad and carries it out from a restaurant that doesn't provide places for people to eat their to-go orders, he shouldn't be required to pay sales tax.

I'm sure that he's also researching this material, and will no doubt have some brilliant idea about how to turn it into another moneymaking proposition.

It's now Wednesday afternoon again and in a little while Suzi and the dog will be driving her e-cart over to Schwartzi's house for another session of magic, or whatever business they're planning. After an extended effort, I get her to promise me she'll drive that cart of hers on the sidewalks as much as possible.

I see that the kid left a message for me.

Peter:
Next time you see Marian, please tell her that we would appreciate her not interrupting our Wednesday afternoon appointments with Mister Schwartz, to serve us tea.

Damn! Her Asian Boy spy network must have operatives in every restaurant in the Marina. I should have known I couldn't keep anything from her. Now that we've been 'outed,' it may mean that we can use the boat instead of the Foghorn Motel.

They just left a few minutes ago and I'm watching the afternoon news. Half way through the broadcast I see that my ex-wife is going to be interviewed. The newscaster announces her.

"We're here on the Peninsula in Marina del Rey with District Attorney Myra Scot, who has been called to the scene. Miss District Attorney, can you tell us anything about this situation?"

Myra looks as beautiful as ever, even though she's darkened her flame-red hair and now wears it in a bun, to go along with her school-marm style of politically correct wardrobe.

"Our office has been informed that the owner of this residence, a Mister Robert Balscomb, may have been shot to death in his den. We haven't been able to gain access to the murder scene yet because of security devices in effect, but a local magician named the Great Schwartzi is definitely someone we consider to be a 'person of interest' we would like to interview. If the magician is still locked in the room with the victim, when we get in there, he will be thoroughly questioned.

We've gotten cooperation from the company who built the secure room and their 'entry' crew is now using blowtorches to cut through the steel door so we can get inside that room."

That's enough for me to hear. I know exactly where the kid is going and I also know that my Hummer can get there first. Myra said that Schwartzi might still be in the safe-room with Balscomb's body, but I'm not taking any chances. I'm going to beat Suzi to Schwartzi's place and make sure that if he's there, she doesn't go anywhere near him.

What am I thinking? How can he be there? He's locked in the safe-room with Balscomb's body. I don't care. I'm going over to his place anyway. He said he was working on a plan to get in and out of that room, and I'm a devout believer in the magic of illusions.

I'm not worried about a speeding ticket because if any local cop stops me, he's probably a customer of Murray's Chinese restaurant, and all I'll have to do is mention Suzi's name and the fact that she may be going into harm's way and I'll get a siren escort all the way to wherever she is.

I see her e-cart riding towards Schwartzi's house. It's about block away, but I'm going much faster than she is because I'm on the street and she's driving on the sidewalk. As I approach Schwartzi's place I see several squad cars parked there with their light bars activated. I guess Myra didn't want to take any chances either, even though she probably still believes that the magician is locked in that safe-room with the victim.

As I pull up to the house I see a yellow blanket covering something up on the street. Just then Suzi arrives and walks over to the cop in charge, who she obviously knows. I can't hear what they're talking about, but I see a tear running down her cheek as she hugs the dog. The cop recognizes me and realizes that I'm with the kid, so he feels safe in talking to me.

"What's the problem here officer?"

"Like I just told your little girl, there was a traffic accident here. A hit-and-run driver killed a pedestrian who lives in this house. The neighbors say he's some old magician."

46

4

This is a terrible situation. I feel sorry for the kid, because it's not the first time she's lost someone close to her. It happened with her mother, then her stepfather and then again last year when a detective sergeant dock neighbor we represented had a terminal illness.

There's nothing I can say. Myra came over and spent almost an hour with her, but it's going to take time for her to get over it this time.

Before Myra left I was able to sit down with her and get some of the remarkable details of the Balscomb case. All the facts that the authorities have come from statements made by Balscomb's housekeeper Marian and his nephew Jessie, and are as follow:

After they all rode with the nephew to an ophthalmologist appointment where his eyes were examined for glasses and then dilated, Balscomb, Jessie and Marian stopped for some groceries and then returned to their residence. When arriving home, Balscomb noticed that Jessie was dozing in the back seat, so he suggested that Marian let Jessie continue to relax in the car while she brought the groceries inside and put them away. Balscomb went upstairs to his room and Marian went back outside, woke up Jessie and led him inside. A little while later Balscomb asked Jessie to call the Great Schwartzi to come over and visit for a while. Jessie couldn't see the numbers on the phone because of his recent dilation, so Marian called the magician and invited him over. Jessie confirmed this because he heard Marian using the hall telephone, just outside of his room.

While they were waiting for Schwartzi to arrive, Balscomb asked Marian to give him a back rub. Marian then told Jessie that if Schwartzi comes while the back rub is still in progress, that Jessie should go downstairs and open the door for him. Jessie agreed, and then went back to his room, which was next door to his uncle's room.

A few minutes later the phone in Jessie's room rang. It was Marian. She asked him to please get his hourglass and leave it on the hallway table outside his uncle's room. Jessie had an old one in his room and used it occasionally to time his game playing on the computer. He was told

49

that Schwartzi requested that it be available when he arrived there.

Jessie thought the hourglass was on a table near his door, but even with his still blurry vision he was able to discover that it had been moved during house cleaning and was now on top of his dresser, on the other side of the room. Per Marian's request, Jessie put the hourglass out on the hall table.

About ten minutes later the doorbell rang and Jessie didn't see or hear Marian going to answer it, so also as requested, he went downstairs and opened the front door. Even with his blurry vision he could tell it was Schwartzi because there was no mistaking his bushy head of hair and full beard.

Jessie told Schwartzi that he should go upstairs to Balscomb's room. Schwartzi grunted an acknowledgement and followed Jessie up the stairs. As Jessie entered his room he saw Schwartzi pick up the hourglass off of the hall table and walk over to Balscomb's room, at which time he knocked several times on the door before opening it and walking in.

As Balscomb's door was closing, Jessie heard Marian greet Schwartzi and apologize for not coming down to meet him as he came in.

About fifteen or twenty minutes later, Marian left Balscomb and Schwartzi in the room together and went downstairs to prepare some sandwiches and refreshments for them. On the way, she passed by Jessie's room and asked him if he wanted anything from the kitchen. He declined her offer.

Shortly thereafter, Marian returned from the kitchen carrying a tray with the requested refreshments. After knocking on Balscomb's door, she discovered that the doorknob lock was set and she could not enter the room. She knocked again, but there was no response. She told Jessie about this and they were both very concerned, so they used an emergency master key and opened the door. To their surprise, they found that the steel security door had slid down behind it and was locked in place. This meant that one of the room's 'panic' buttons was activated, so the suite's door automatically slammed down and the security service was immediately notified.

The steel door to Balscomb's safe-suite has an approximate six-inch diameter round ship-style porthole in it. It can be completely closed from the inside with a steel shutter, but it wasn't, and through the translucent cover plate both Marian and

51

Jesse were able to make out some shadows in the room. What they saw chilled their blood, because it was the shadow of Schwartzi slightly moving and holding a gun in his hand. Then the doorbell rang and Marian went downstairs to let the two security guards in.

Marian and the security men went back upstairs and they all looked through the portlight and saw the same shadowy figure waving the handgun. They also pounded on the door and shouted at the people inside, but it was useless because of the safe-room's soundproofing.

Less than a minute later everything in the room went dark. The regular police were called and quickly responded, but they also couldn't break through the security door.

It was over an hour before the company that installed the safe-room arrived with their entry crew. While they were working with their blowtorches, Myra was outside making her statement to the press.

"That's interesting Myra, but why haven't I seen these details in the newspapers or on television? This seems like a really juicy story, and one that you could probably get a lot of miles out of. I know that Schwartzi was found dead outside of his house later that afternoon, so why the hell did you cut him loose and let him go home?"

She doesn't answer me. Something's wrong here.

"C'mon, hon. Tell me why you released him."

After another minute of silence she looks up at me like a confused kid.

"We didn't release him. We never had him. When we finally broke through the door, went in and searched the room, Mr. Schwartz was not there."

5

I enjoy an occasional surprise, but this one takes the cake. "What do you mean he wasn't in there? Marian called to invite him over, Jessie went downstairs and let him in and he followed Jessie upstairs and then went into the room. When he went in the room, Marian said hello to him. Jessie's room is only a few feet down the hallway from Balscomb's, and heard it all. Balscomb didn't have any windows in his room that the magician could've used to escape.

"No one passed by Jessie's room after Marian went down to the kitchen. By this time Jessie's eyes had almost cleared up and he surely would have noticed if the magician had walked past his room... and even if Schwartzi did manage to sneak past Jessie's room he would probably have bumped into Marian as she was returning from the kitchen. I can't believe he wasn't there. Did you search the room thoroughly?"

"Peter, I had the best CSI crew in town with me. They went over that room and the entire house with a fine-tooth comb. There was no sign of Schwartzi. Only Balscomb, with one bullet in his chest. The gun was still there and it had Schwartzi's fingerprints on it, but there was no Schwartzi."

"Wait a minute, Miss District Attorney. If that room was all locked up, how did Marian get out when she went to the kitchen?"

"It wasn't locked when she left the room. Either Schwartzi or Balscomb must have hit one of the panic buttons after she exited. There are three buttons like that located in the suite, and it's impossible for someone to push the button and then escape because each button is about ten feet from the nearest door, and those steel slide-downs drop in less than one second after a button is pushed. And another thing that definitely places him in the suite when the gun went off was all the witnesses seeing him standing there holding the gun."

"The suite? What do you mean the suite? I thought it was just a safe room."

"Not quite. It's more than that. Money was obviously no object with Balscomb, so when he had the house built he specified that his bedroom, private bathroom and adjoining den all be one large safe-suite. That way, in the event that it was necessary for him to be locked in there for a period of time, he would have access to sleeping quarters and plumbing. A small refrigerator in the den contained emergency food supplies. He even succeeded in getting a variance from the building department to avoid their window requirements. Our office has a complete inventory of the items we found, along with mucho pictures taken. If you want, you can pull a Sherlock Holmes routine and solve this thing for us."

"Isn't there at least one person on the entire District Attorney's investigation staff that has a theory as to what really happened, or will it be left up to us to solve this case?"

"No one in our office can explain it Peter, so that's why we put out an APB for the magician. I figured that when we caught up with him he'd want to alibi himself out that room before the victim got shot, so he would be encouraged to fill in some blanks for us... but he got run over instead, and now we'll never know what happened.

"As far as our office is concerned, this is a closed case. Schwartzi did it and then escaped, only to get hit by a car later that same afternoon.

"We're not giving out any more details other than the fact that we had a suspect and several independent eye witnesses to the crime. The press has theorized that we arrested Schwartzi at the scene, but being a professional magician, he managed to get out of his handcuffs and escaped from our custody and hurried home, where he was then hit by a motorist and killed. All we've been giving them is the standard 'we can't comment during an open investigation.' We haven't made any attempts to rebut their theories, so as far as the press is concerned they've got it all figured out – and if the press and the public are both happy with it, then so are we. Case closed."

She's had enough conversation with me for today, and I think it's a little tough for her to display any deficiency of her investigation to an ex-husband she never really respected that much. As she starts to leave the boat I notice two pairs of eyes peering out from behind the slightly open foreward stateroom door. The human ones look concerned, so I do a little performance for them. Maybe it'll get me a few points with the kid.

"How nice for you. One guy gets shot to death, another gets run down and killed, and your office closes the case because you can't figure it out. You guys just don't care because there's no one to prosecute. What is probably the most intriguing double homicide of the century goes down on your turf and you aren't even looking into it. You disappoint me."

Nothing. She steps off the boat with a goodbye wave and tells me to take care of the kid and that she'll be calling her later this evening. She then turns around and gives me some advice.

"And by the way Peter, if I were you I'd stay away from that maid for while. We don't want you tampering with a prosecution witness."

"Tampering?"

"Well, I'd prefer using that word instead of another right now."

That does it. I now realize it is absolutely impossible for me to do anything in Los Angeles County without Suzi and the District Attorney knowing about it. I no longer have any privacy. Between Suzi and Myra, my life is an open book. And I definitely don't consider what I've been planning on doing to Marian as 'tampering.'

The most interesting thing I heard Myra say was that Marian was a possible witness. Not a suspect, but a witness. I guess the District Attorney's office doesn't know that Balscomb was worth a tenth of a billion dollars, because with that much money involved, both Marian and the nephew would be more than just witnesses.

When I turn around there is a small audience waiting for me in the main saloon. She's got that serious look on her face, but as usual, doesn't say anything. I look down at her.

"What is it now? You don't think I shouldn't have talked to her like that?"

"What are you going to do about this case Peter?"

"Why should I do anything about it? He was your magic teacher. I never even met the guy. You heard your friend Myra. You know as much about this case as I do. If you want it solved, then go solve it yourself. You're the genius around here." The dynamic duo exits without further comment.

As much as I hate to admit it, Myra is right. I'd like to believe it's a little bit of jealousy on her part, but that would only be wishful thinking. I know the kid is no fan of Marian for one main reason: any woman I find myself attracted to presents a threat to Suzi's master plan of getting Myra and I back together. Whatever their reasons may be, I know that I'll have to cool it with Marian, so I call her to express my condolences for the loss of her employer. She reluctantly agrees with me about holding off on getting together until this whole mess is over.

Now I know why women call all of us men dogs. It's because in the back of my mind, I can't keep thinking about taking advantage of the fact that her boss has been whacked and that now she may need a place to sleep.

Stuart is calling. Probably to tell me that he found out about the law regarding sales tax on carryout food.

"Hi Stu. Did you do your homework?"

"You bet I did Pete. I went to the Valley's Board of Equalization's office and got all the information I needed."

"Let's see, as a wild guess I'd say that section 6359 covers it. Am I close?"

"Ha. You're a clever one. I see that you checked things out too. That's a complicated section, and some of it depends on whether or not eighty percent of the seller's gross receipts are from the sale of food products... information that no outsider has access to."

"Stuart I'm going to give you some very valuable advice now. It may be worth a lot of money to you in the near future."

"Okay, I'm listening. What's the advice Pete?"

"Move on."

That's it? Move on?"

"You got it pal. Don't waste your time obsessing over the minutia of whether or not some restaurant is making an extra few percentage points by skimming sales tax. From what you've told me, the receipt they gave you indicated an amount of sales tax was collected. In order for that designation to appear on a cash register printed receipt, it means that the amount of tax collected is being accounted for, and that means they're probably paying it to the state.

"In the time you'll spend trying to stir up trouble and avoiding paying a dollar here and there, you can probably start up a new business and make enough money to buy one of the restaurants you're complaining about."

Stuart grudgingly agrees and promises to take my advice, but the thought of money raises another question, so I write a quick note, shake the dog-biscuit box and send a dog-mail to the foreward stateroom. If I remember correctly, the kid mentioned that she was considering a business deal with the Great Schwartzi. He's dead now, and I'm wondering if she's involved in anything that needs cleaning up. She's pretty tight with her money, so I doubt if she let that old man get any of it. Just to play safe, I might as well do my duty as her legal guardian and at least inquire if she needs any legal help.

My note to her is a simple question that asks:

Did you give any money to the magician? And if so, how much?

It takes a while before my answer comes back. About ten minutes have passed and I hear the large paws approaching. I remove the message from his collar and look at it in disbelief. It contains only two words:

Fifty thousand.

6

How the hell did she get her little hands on fifty grand? I know she does some outside consulting work, but that's a pretty nice piece of change to stash on the side. I check our online account status at the bank to see if there's been any withdrawal of funds from her trust account, and there it is. A fifty thousand dollar withdrawal was made just one or two days after she started taking her magic lessons.

I'm the trustee on that account and I'm supposed to have knowledge of and approve any substantial withdrawals. How could this have happened? There are several million of her dollars in accounts at that bank, so we get some respect when we call there, and that's exactly what I'm doing now.

After being passed around from one executive to another I finally get connected with the head of their trust department and am told that when the accounts were originally set up, the paperwork indicated that the law firm was the official trustee and that I was a managing partner of the law firm. This means that she is the other managing partner and has the same access to the money that I do. It also means that I'm just a figurehead and the kid knew it all the time because she prepared the paperwork when the accounts were opened.

I can't believe it. She's always two steps ahead of me. If Schwartz had been killed and I hadn't checked with the bank, I would have never found out these details about the accounts.

After thinking it over for a while, I cool down. After all, it's her money and she should have the right to do whatever she wants with it, barring some stupid expenditure that would only be a complete waste. At this time I have no idea what the business she invested in was, and for all I know it might have even wound up being a huge moneymaker.

The only thing to do now is try to get some information out of the kid to see what the whole story is and what can be done to get that money back for her. This will require some very delicate questioning and must be done by a professional. I press a button on my speed-dial.

"What is it now Sherlock? I'm on my way back to the office. Have you solved the mystery already?"

"Suzi gave fifty large to the magician."

"What?"

"You heard me. The kid gave fifty thousand dollars to the Great Schwartzi, just two days after they met at her friend's birthday party."

"Why?"

"I have no idea."

"Did you ask her?"

"Myra, I'm sure you realize that my rapport with her isn't what I'd like it to be. I've never been able to deal with kids. They intimidate me, especially this one. You mentioned that you were going to speak to her this evening, so I thought that maybe you could get some information out of her. She looks up to you."

"I can't believe it Peter, stooping lower than I thought was possible. You want me to exploit my friendship with her strictly for investigative purposes... to mislead her into thinking that a friendly conversation isn't a cross-examination. You are low."

"Okay, miss holier-than-thou, why not just tell her that we'll all go to dinner this evening at Pollo Meshuga? We can meet you there - and I'm buying."

"See you at seven, Petey."

During our marriage there were very few things we both enjoyed doing at the same time, but eating a Pollo Meshuga was one of them. Not only is the food pretty good, but they also make a dynamite Patrón Margarita and usually have at least four large screen television sets tuned in to a Spanish-language soccer game somewhere in the world.

Not being bi-lingual, I never understand the play-by-play. The only thing I know for sure is when someone scores, because the announcer goes crazy with one of his trademark shouts of "goooooaaaaall!"

Another message is sent to the foreward stateroom telling her that the three of us are going out for dinner tonight because Myra wants to ask her for some advice about the Balscomb murder, and our departure time will be at 18:45 hours. She knows what that means, because it's 'cop talk.' I don't expect any argument this time, because she really likes Myra and secretly wants to get us back together again, so that she can be adopted. I've never discussed it with her, but Myra and I both get the feeling that she has some master plan toward that end result. I try not to think about it too much because I'm afraid that as far as Myra's concerned, it's a dead issue. She's had enough of me to last her a lifetime. The kid doesn't know any better yet.

At 6:45 the two of are them waiting for me on the boarding steps. She's already put the dog's Doggles on him, so he knows he's going for a ride. Doggles are special aviator-style goggles designed specifically to protect a dog's eyes from damage while riding in a vehicle with his head sticking out in the wind.

When we get into my yellow Hummer the dog automatically rides shotgun and sits up in the front passenger seat with his huge head sticking up and out of the open sunroof. The kid sits in the back seat, from where she feels free to constantly issue driving directions to me. As we cruise down the street toward the restaurant we get the usual looks from pedestrians and other motorists, because with the Doggles on and his large ears flapping in the wind, Bernie looks like some World War I air ace. We've even nicknamed him the Brown Baron. Whoever has a camera handy always tries to get a shot as we pass by.

It's ten minutes later and we're approaching the restaurant. The car-parking guys have spotted us and all three of them are in position and waiting. When we pull up, one opens my door, another places a milk crate on the ground to help Suzi negotiate the large step down out of vehicle, and the third one opens the dog's door, removes the Doggles and leads him to the rear service entrance of the restaurant, where he will wait for us while he plays with the restaurant owner's cat. They've become friends over the past year or so.

I have a suspicion that the cat is really being used as a form of vermin control, which is okay with me. But if I ever find out that the cat is no longer around, I won't be ordering any of their chicken dishes for a while.

We walk in the front door and see that Myra is already sitting at our favorite semi-circular booth, working on her first Patrón Margarita. Now that the county provides her with a car and driver, she doesn't hesitate to imbibe socially. Suzi slides in right next to her so that she'll be seated between us.

I really have to hand it to my ex-wife. She's sharp as a tack. I neglected to tell her that Suzi thinks she was invited to help out with the Balscomb case, but during the first twenty minutes of the kid's questioning her, I see that she's playing along perfectly. The kid asks some questions that never occurred to me.

We're almost finished with the main course and the fifty thousand dollar subject hasn't yet been raised. I'm starting to wonder how Myra's going to gently slide it into the conversation.

I get my answer when the flan is brought out.

"Suzi, while our investigators were going through the personal papers of your magician friend, we found some notations he made about owing you some money. Is there anything to that? I mean, was he going to refund you some of the money you were paying for lessons or something? Ordinarily I wouldn't ask, but as you know, it is part of a murder investigation, and knowing how you dislike being subpoenaed, I thought that maybe you could tell me what that money memo was about."

Suzi thinks for a second and realizes her inescapable position of being completely surrounded by two adults who want to get some information out of her. There's no doing an about-face and marching away this time. She looks up at Myra.

"I suppose he already told you about the money."

"He may have mentioned it, but I'd really like to hear it from you. His credibility isn't that great with me."

Smart... she's playing 'nice cop.' That doesn't leave a very desirable roll for me to play, so I think I'll just keep my mouth shut and let Myra do the heavy lifting here.

"I invested fifty thousand dollars with the late Mister Schwartz. It was to help him design some special illusions for a couple of big-name celebrity magicians that appear on television and in Las Vegas. He showed me the contracts he had with them guaranteeing that he would receive almost two hundred thousand dollars when the tricks were delivered. He explained the illusions to me and how they worked, and I thought it was doable, so I lent him the money."

Nothing gets past Myra.

"Suzi honey, at first you said you 'invested' the money, but then you said you 'lent it to him.' Those two words mean quite different things... so which one was it?"

"Well, it was like kind of both. It was part investment because I was to get a percentage of the profits over and above the investment. But it was also like a loan, because I was given some collateral to hold."

Her mention of collateral comes as a complete surprise, but also strengthens my opinion about the kid's business acumen. Myra keeps a cool demeanor and continues with her conversational interrogation.

"Oh, that's nice. I always thought you were a good little businessperson, but this really shows how good you are. What type of collateral did he give you?"

"I'm really not supposed to say. It was given to me in confidence."

"Suzi, when you take your courses at Harvard Law School I think you'll learn that there's no magician-student privilege"

The kid doesn't take that remark very kindly and she lets Myra know about it.

"I'm quite aware of the various privileges one can assert, and I know that an official one didn't exist between Mister Schwartz and me, but I promised him that I wouldn't say anything, so it's a matter of honor with me, not a legal privilege to rely on."

She's got a good point there and Myra knows it. This isn't a courtroom, it's a restaurant, so Myra may have been a little out of line with her sarcastic remark about privileges. It's also obvious that neither one of us is going to get any more information about that collateral out of her, so Myra wisely gives up on trying and tries to change the subject.

"Okay, I can respect your promise to him, but keep in mind that he's still a likely murderer. Now, have you solved our locked-room mystery yet?"

I think I detect some trace of a smile on Suzi's face as she answers.

"I haven't got it figured out yet, but I do have some ideas. Can you let me look at the scene of the crime? Is it still secure? I mean, has anything been moved or changed since you were up there last?"

This is also a surprise to both of us. Can it be that the kid really has a theory about the Balscomb murder case? Myra keeps her cool.

"Sure. I can arrange for you to go over there tomorrow afternoon. Should I have someone pick you up?"

"No, that won't be necessary. My assistant will be coming with, so we'll go in his van. And he would also like to see Mister Schwartz' body."

Myra looks at me with a questioning expression on her face, but by my blank look she can tell that I don't know what the kid means either. She did mention that her assistant will be driving a van and the only person we know that has one who might also be interested in seeing a dead body is Victor Gutierrez, from the well-known firm, 1800AUTOPSY. Myra agrees to let the assistant see Schwartz' body as long as Suzi stays in the morgue's visitor waiting room. She may be a good little detective, but she's still just a kid, and the County's autopsy room isn't the place for her, no matter how smart she is.

On our way out of the restaurant Myra calls me aside while Suzi is fetching her beast.

"Did you take my advice?"

"About what?"

"About diddling that maid. Remember? I warned you about that."

"Oh yeah. Well, it may please you to know that I'm still celibate. We've decided to wait until you've solved the case before we get back together again, so I guess my sex life will be on hiatus for some time."

"Sure it will, big boy, if you stay off that houseboat too."

Now I have some idea how celebrities must feel, hounded by paparazzi, living in a fishbowl.

Last night's dinner conversation hasn't cleared much up for me. I still don't know how Balscomb got killed, or who did it, or if Schwartz' death is connected to it. If there's one thing that crime solvers would rather not see, it's a coincidence – and both Balscomb and Schwartz becoming dead on the same afternoon is a real humdinger of one. I'll have to think about that. At least I was correct in suspecting who Suzi's van-driving assistant is, because Victor just stepped onto the boat. After we chat for a few minutes the kid and dog both let him know that they're ready to visit the crime scene.

Shortly after they leave the boat I sit down to watch the afternoon news and learn of a new development. The Balscomb family, which consists of his nephew Jessie, has retained the services of an attorney named Morris Arthur, who is reportedly a former law professor. They will be bringing a civil action against the estate of the Great Schwartzi for damages due to the intentional causing of Mister Balscomb's death.

That lawyer's name sounds vaguely familiar to me, but I can't remember why. The bringing of this action is really nothing out of the ordinary, because every crime is also an actionable tort. Victims don't usually waste their time and money bringing civil actions against criminals because most of them are incarcerated and judgment proof. There are some exceptions, one well-known one being the civil action for wrongful death brought against O.J. Simpson by the family of one of the murder victims.

In that particular case the defendant Simpson was acquitted by a criminal court but that didn't stop the family, because in civil cases a unanimous jury verdict isn't required. The 'beyond a reasonable doubt' standard of proof only exits in criminal trials. I think that both the criminal and the civil juries in the O.J. Simpson affair basically thought the same thing: 'he *probably* did it.' 'Probably' isn't good enough in a criminal case, but is sufficient in a civil case. Simpson won the criminal case and lost the civil one.

If the Balscomb murder was ever brought to trial the prosecution might not have been able to prove that Schwartz was guilty beyond a reasonable doubt because they never found him at the scene. But with the testimony of four people, plus the fingerprints on the gun, a civil jury would probably be convinced that it's very likely Schwartz was involved in Balscomb's death, and that's enough for a civil jury to bring in a judgment for the plaintiff.

I hope the kid doesn't get sucked into this controversy, because she doesn't do very well under subpoena. She either wants to run the show herself or not go to court at all.

Victor brings the kid and dog back to the boat, but as usual, no report is made to me about any findings. I notice that she's carrying a magnifying glass, but that must be a prop to put her into the 'detective' mode. I'm surprised she isn't wearing one of those double-ended deerstalker caps like Holmes used to wear.

The Asian Boys deliver our dinner, but tonight it's not from the Chinese restaurant. Instead, it was picked up at a local Italian restaurant and includes my favorites: eggplant parmigiana and antipasto with anchovies. They even brought some spumoni for dessert.

After dinner the kid requests a meeting, at which time she informs me that we have a new client.

"Peter, I want you to represent Mister Schwartz's interests."

"Are you talking about the late Mister Schwartz?"

She nods affirmatively. This gives me a chance to use the only Chinese word I know in a sentence. "That's *sonchingping!*"

I get a startled look out of her. Even the dog looks at me in amazement that I know the Chinese word for 'crazy.' "Suzi, it's tough enough handling live clients. I can't represent Schwartz. He's dead."

"He's still going to be put on trial. The Balscomb family is suing his estate for wrongful death."

"So? What's the problem? We don't have anything to do with that. And besides, who has standing to retain our firm to represent the late Mister Schwartz? We can't just jump into a lawsuit because he was your teacher. We need someone to request our services."

"Okay. I'm making the request."

"How can you do that? You aren't a member of his family."

"I do have standing, because I'm a creditor. His estate owes me fifty thousand dollars plus interest. If the Balscomb suit is successful it'll wipe out whatever assets that Schwartz had and my creditor's claim will be defeated."

She's got a good point there. I look down at the dog, hoping he understood my recent lecture about the double job required in certain cases. This is one of them, because in order to defeat the Balscomb family claim against the Schwartz estate, I'll have to also conduct a criminal defense case on Schwartz' behalf. That defense will have to create reasonable doubt in the minds of the jury about him murdering Balscomb.

There's only one problem with this double job. I have no idea how Schwartz got out of that room. And if he didn't do it, I'd better offer the jury another suspect... someone who actually could have gotten into that secure room, shot Balscomb and then got out.

No problem. I tell the kid the terms of my representation.

"First of all, this can't be a law firm matter, because you're a part of the firm. You'll have to retain me privately to represent your interest as a creditor of the estate, and you'll have to pay me a fee to represent you. Secondly, I haven't the slightest idea of how to defend Schwartz or who to point the finger of guilt at if he didn't do it. I'll tell you what: here's my proposal... you figure out the secret of this locked-room mystery and I'll do the courtroom work."

She looks up at me. No comment is forthcoming. After her about-face maneuver and march toward the foreward stateroom, she tosses her closing remark at me: "Deal."

Great. I've got a new client and it's probably the most difficult client any lawyer ever had. I also have no affirmative defense, no witnesses, no facts, no theory and no argument. Aside from that, the case is pretty solid. I hope she doesn't expect me to handle this on a contingency, because as far as I can see it's on an express route to the dumper... and with the publicity that a case like this will probably attract, it'll no doubt take my illustrious career along with it. Myra's going to love watching me go down in flames with this one.

The way it looks now, the only way to get Schwartz off of the hook is to put someone else on it. Let's see... the usual things you look for are motive, means and opportunity. In this case it looks like no one in particular had any special motive to see Balscomb dead. As for means, it could be anyone able to get in and out of a completely sealed off safe-room. Same goes for opportunity. Hmmmn... welcome back to square one, Peter.

I'm bothered by something the kid told me. Why on earth would Balscomb's nephew go through the time and aggravation of suing Schwartz' estate for wrongful death? Sure, they might get an award of a couple of hundred thousand dollars if they're successful, but when you've already got a tenth of a billion bucks, why waste your time and energy for chickenfeed like a wrongful death suit? There's probably some other agenda I don't know about yet, but I'm sure it's only a matter of time before it becomes apparent.

I've worked on this case long enough today, so it's time for my afternoon break and a look at what passes for news, locally.

After the usual items about last night's car chases, car-jackings and other 'if-it-bleeds-it-leads' items, the blow-dried anchor people let us know that they have a late-breaking exclusive. Their crime reporter appears on the screen, standing in front of the Marina del Rey Sheriff's office.

"We have just obtained a copy of the police report filed on the murder of Robert Balscomb, and the witness statements it contains create a mystery the likes of which this reporter has never seen before. It seems that Mister Balscomb was killed while locked inside the very expensive, safe, panic-room that he had installed when his house was custom built for him. At least four eyewitnesses, including two private security officers, have signed affidavits to the fact that they were able to look through a small translucent window opening and see what they believed to be another person waving a gun at the victim.

"When the safe-room manufacturer's entry crew finally got the door open, the police found only the victim. The person who shot him was not in the room. Witness statements report that the other person who reportedly was in the room with the victim was none other than the well-known magician the Great Schwartzi, who was admitted to the victim's home earlier that day and spent time with him in the safe-room. Schwartzi was found later in front of his own residence, the victim of a fatal hit-and-run accident caused by a vehicle that has yet to be found, and the police are requesting the public's assistance in this matter. At this point in time, there is no explanation as to how the magician managed to escape from the Balscomb safe-room.

"One of our sources at the downtown courthouse informs us that the Balscomb estate has filed a multi-million dollar legal action against the estate of the Great Schwartzi, and we've also learned that the Schwartzi estate will be defended by Marina del Rey attorney Peter Sharp, who represents a creditor of that estate."

The reporter then turns it back over to the studio, and the anchor people continue by filling the public in on the details of both deceased gentlemen, where they were born, and whatever non-interesting details they could dig up.

It had to happen sooner or later because juicy stuff like this never remains quiet too long before being discovered. It's a good thing that Myra's office kept its mouth shut and didn't make any comments before now. They probably realized it would hit the fan pretty soon and they didn't want to have to defend anything they might have previously said on camera.

I've just changed the message on our answering machine to say that our law firm has no statement to make. That should take care of the phone calls we'll no doubt be getting from reporters all over the country. If anyone wants to get in touch with us they can do it by email. The only calls we'll be accepting are from people who know our private cell phone numbers. One good thing about this mess is now that I'm officially on the case, I can add Jack Bibber-man's prior Balscomb investigation fees onto the bill and the kid will pay for it out of her proceeds from the estate... if there are any.

A dog-mail comes in reminding me that I promised to fill in as a substitute lecturer at B.L.'s Bar Review Seminar this evening.

Bart Levin is a former law professor of mine who now conducts a review class for unaccredited law school students who must take and pass the First Year Law Students' Examination, which has been nicknamed the 'Baby Bar.' Once having passed this exam, those students will then be permitted to continue on with their studies and after graduation, take the regular Bar exam. This test was instituted many years ago to weed out the people who would never have a chance to pass the Bar exam, and save a lot of people years of studying in vain.

In the past I've done some lecturing at Bart's seminars and promised him that I'd be available to fill in if one of his regulars was unavailable. This evening I'll be taking over for another lawyer who is busy preparing for a big trial, and Bart has assured me that no lecture preparation will be necessary because I'm simply to go over some past criminal law Bar exam questions with the class.

The classes are being held in the evening school section of a local high school, and the students look exactly like the ones who attended my unaccredited night law school over twenty years ago. Their ages range from the twenties through the seventies, and include everyone from housewives to surgeons.

This evening's selection of criminal law questions includes several that are designed to determine whether or not a student taking the test has the ability to find all the possible crimes that can be charged in a given factual situation. This is a lot like some cartoon-like drawings on the back of frosted cereal boxes that challenge children to try and find all the hidden numbers in the picture.

Strangely enough, the students who do the worst on these criminal law questions are the police officers. It seems that they have a great difficulty in transitioning from the mindset used on the street to the one required in the classroom. As many people have learned, quite often the police will be reluctant to get involved in minor disputes between domestic partners, neighbors or landlords and tenants, suggesting that "this looks like a civil matter between you people... consult with a lawyer."

That might be okay out there in real life, but a Bar exam is nothing like reality. The person answering the question can't refer people to a civil lawyer. Every possible issue involving the criminal law must be discussed, whether it would be important enough to warrant an arrest or not.

We finish up with the questions, and as usual there are always a couple of hangers-on who have some questions or comments for me. I really enjoy this interaction with the students, because in some ways it takes me back to those enjoyable nights when I was in their position.

All the students have gone now with the exception of one dapper gentleman who surprises me.

"Mister Sharp, I know this hasn't anything to do with our class this evening, but I happen to be a professional magician, and I couldn't help but be interested in the matters surrounding the death of the Great Schwartzi. I saw on the news that you're involved in that case, and I want you to know that if there's anything I can do to help you out that you shouldn't hesitate to call me."

He hands me his business card and I see that it has the usual magician's logo of a rabbit coming out of a hat. His professional name is Michael Brody.

"Thank you Mister Brody, but shouldn't your name end in an 'i,' and have a 'great' preceding it?"

"Well, maybe that was the way to go twenty or thirty years ago, but it's looked at as being a little corny nowadays, so I just go with my regular name."

"Honesty is always refreshing to discover. Did you know the late Mister Schwartz?"

"Never had the pleasure, but I've read some of his books. I understand that at one time he was quite the man in the world of magic."

"What happened? Did he forget how to do the tricks?"

"No, but professional bookers are looking for someone with flash. Someone who can excite an audience and keep their attention. Someone who the people might want to believe is having an affair with his beautiful long-legged assistant. After performing professionally for over forty years, I guess that Mister Schwartz decided to stop trying to be flashy and just wanted to create illusions for other guys. In a way, he really became a magicians' magician. From what I've heard, he was very highly regarded by the whole profession."

This is nice to hear, but it's been a long day for me, so I might as well draw this conversation to a close by finding out if Mister Brody has the right stuff or not.

"Mister Brody, you're a professional magician. You've probably followed all the details of this case and know about Schwartz visiting that secure room and supposedly getting out of it after the steel door slammed shut, so tell me. What's your take on this whole thing? How did Schwartz get out of that room?"

His answer is an interesting one, and leads me to believe that he'll do just fine when he takes his regular Bar exam a few years from now.

"Mister Sharp, Schwartz didn't get out of that room. Magicians don't do the impossible: they're human beings, just like the rest of us. Everything that we do is really quite simple... we just try to make it look like we did something impossible.

"From what I understand, your little girl had been taking some magic lessons with Schwartz, and I'm sure he explained that to her while showing her the basics of some of our standard tricks.

"If you want to solve this case I'd suggest that you look for as simple an answer as possible and leave the complicated theories to others."

His answer doesn't help me very much, but I know that he's right, and Suzi probably knows it too. I think that the locked room aspect of this case is just a red herring to misdirect us from what really took place. I've explained this in previous lectures to the students while showing them some Bar questions that tried to cloud the issues by trying to create some sympathy for someone desperately in need. The standard rule in answering Bar questions is to 'watch out for widows and orphans.' You must analyze each question on its own merits, no matter how much you'd like to see a sympathetic person win.

I'm going to have to practice what I preach now, because this problem should be solved the old fashion way. Any time there's a high-profile murder case it's always a good idea to look for a trail left by either love or money. In this case I don't think that love played much of a part, so I might as well follow the money... who has it, how much, and where it will now go. I call Jack Bibberman and have him continue with his investigation by widening it to include financial information and who is supposed to inherit from both dead guys. I already know about Balscomb's huge fortune, which will probably go to his nephew, but I don't really think there's much to look for in Schwartz' estate.

Suzi managed to get a copy of the report prepared by the LAPD's Traffic Accident Division, so she can start to look for the hit-and-run driver that ran down her magic teacher. I took a quick look at it and noticed that she highlighted the part where it said there were no recent skid marks found at the scene. This could mean that the driver didn't see Schwartz and just plowed right into him... or that it was an intentional rundown. The problem with the latter murder scenario is that I can't think of a motive. There might be some nut out there who might think Schwartz stole a magic trick or illusion from him, but other than private parties and the children's hospital, Schwartz hasn't performed publicly in so many years that the revenge motive is unlikely.

There's no use my visiting the crime scene because that would do me about as much good as lifting the hood of my car if the engine ever unexpectedly died on me. I'll never know why people do that. I did it only once and all I discovered was that the engine was still there. I'd probably learn even less from the crime scene. To me, crime scenes are a lot like a football game: you can see it a lot better on television than you can by going there. Suzi will no doubt talk Myra into letting her see the D.A.'s file on this case, and it'll contain all the pictures I need to see of that scene.

I've already driven over to Schwartz' house, but I guess that seeing Balscomb's place would be in order, even though it would be an act of futility. The exclusive Peninsula area is only a few blocks away from our boat and it's a beautiful day so I think I'll walk over there. They've done a nice job of building a small neighborhood of multi-million dollar three-story homes here, but they have no back yards and are only about two feet apart from each other. I guess that's the only way to economically do it on such valuable land near the ocean.

Balscomb's house is the last one on the block and looks like it's probably worth more than the others, especially with the Canal and Ocean views. On the way back to our boat I stop on the corner at a lemonade stand operated by two kids about the same size as Suzi. One of them looks up at me with an announcement.

"If you're a cop, there's no free lemonade. Cops have to pay full price too."

I assure the kids that I'm not a cop and leave a full dollar on their table, and walk away without asking for any change. The lemonade is refreshing, but a little too sweet for my taste. As I leave with my drink, the stand's proprietors make sure to let me know where the trashcans are in the direction that I'm walking.

The only other people I'd really like to talk to now are the ones that built and installed Balscomb's safe-rooms, because I have a couple of questions for them. I try to get my questions answered over the phone, but am informed that they absolutely refuse to give telephone interviews. If I want any information about their products I'm going to have to personally visit their office in Mount Vernon, New York. This is another added expense on a losing case. I send a dog-mail to the kid's stateroom letting her know that maybe we should try to cut our losses now and avoid spending another couple of thousand for my trip and more investigation.

To my surprise, she pays me a personal visit and makes an announcement.

"I'll be glad to cover your expenses for the trip to that safe-room company."

"Boy, that's a surprise. What's the big deal here? You can write off the loss, and even if we win, there'll probably be no money for you because Schwartz died before he finished those illusions. His estate can't collect on the contract. There will be no two hundred thousand dollars coming in, and his funeral expenses and other debts will probably eat up whatever assets he has."

You still have to win this case"

"Why? Just because you want to try and get some of your money back?"

"No. The money has nothing to do with it."

"Okay, I give up. If it's not the money, then why is winning this case so important to you?"

"Because of Jessie Balscomb's attorney, Morris Arthur."

"You know this guy?"

"Not personally, but he's the one who represented the drunk driver who killed my mother in her car accident. He had the audacity to sue mother claiming that the accident was her fault."

"Suzi, I'm not familiar with that case... your stepfather handled it. I appreciate the fact that you want to believe that your mother wasn't at fault, but since neither one of us was there, I don't know how..."

She cuts me off mid-sentence with her closing tirade.

"Okay, you and Morris Arthur are both right. The accident was my mother's fault. While she was going through a major intersection on a green light, she intentionally caused her car to suddenly move sideways and force her driver's side door into the front end of Morris Arthur's drunk client's car while the automatic camera photographed him speeding through the red light and into my mother's car.

"It was supposed to have been a slam-dunk case for Mister Arthur. He was representing some corporate executive who had the bad luck of being involved in an accident with a female Asian driver... and we all know that they can't drive. Maybe that's why the drunk's insurance company forked over that couple of million to make the case go away. I didn't like Morris Arthur then, and I don't like him now. That's why we have to win."

That answers another question. In many cases a client's actions are driven by the attorney. This becomes evident in domestic relations cases, where mean-spirited attorneys turn what could be an amicable divorce settlement into a battle for every last penny, often using a child's custody as a the final bargaining chip.

In this case, Morris Arthur is involved, and from what Suzi and some other lawyers I know have said, he follows his own agenda and drags the client along with him. It looks like attorneys like Arthur spend their time searching for the clients that will allow them to achieve their own devious goals, and this time Arthur found Jessie Balscomb... and Suzi found me.

The car service will be picking me up in about an hour and my first-class round trip ticket has just been delivered to the boat by our local travel agent. This is in line with the new rule I just created that provides for first-class accommodations on any business flight that requires being in the air more than two hours.

I could probably have gotten one of the kid's cop friends to talk the safe-room people into answering my questions on the phone, but that wouldn't have satisfied the kid, and I haven't been back east in several years, so this will give me a chance to visit an old friend who lives in Buck's County, Pennsylvania. He's thc only tone-deaf person I know of who owns a great collection of classic jazz records; one of those people who always wanted to play music, but just never had the talent.

I never enjoyed flying very much, but by using the air miles I've accumulated from recent air trips to Thailand and Hawaii, I was able to use them to join the Red Carpet Club, an exclusive service that many large airlines provide for their travelers. These clubs offer luxurious lounges where members can relax while waiting for their flights, and enjoy the perks that include sleeping lounges, complimentary beverages, email internet connection and all-around comfort.

Combined with the extra attention of first-class air travel and the early boarding privilege, this is definitely the way to fly. The more than six hour flight will also give me some time to catch up on my reading, and for this trip I'm going through a collection of short stories about locked-room mysteries and other impossible crimes.

There's no reason I should have to depend on a kid to solve this case: I've been around thirty years more than she has, so I should be just as capable of solving this mystery as her.

Being a first-class traveler, I rent a luxury car for my drive to the Secure-Co offices. Walking into their building I get the feeling I'm in a bank vault. The walls look like they're metal, complete with rivets every foot or so. The company president is expecting me and we sit down in his office for our meeting. There are no brochures around anywhere. If you're interested in one of their products, a security consultant meets with you and goes over the architectural plans of your home.

The first thing they want to make sure of is the structural integrity of your residence, because if you want to have your safe-room anywhere above the first floor, the house's construction must be strong enough to support the extra weight.

They make secure rooms of several different levels, but if you only want to protect yourself for a brief amount of time less than six hours, then you get the kind that Balscomb ordered. It is good for attacks from anything less than heavy artillery, is sound-activated and soundproofed to avoid noise harassment. Any time one of the conveniently located panic buttons is activated, the secure steel doors immediately fall down into place and can only be re-opened from the inside. If electric power has been cut off, a back-up chain-operated winch can be used.

Emergency notification of the authorities is automatically done by a dedicated cell-phone that is connected to the steel bars outside the house's windows, sort of an 'On-Star' set-up like many luxury cars have, but for houses. The bars act as an antenna. This provides communication even if the attackers cut the phone lines too.

One interesting thing that the rooms are equipped with is a secret surveillance camera that watches outside the room, so one inside might know when a threat has ended. There's also a 'black box' that records events like date and exact time of panic button activation, temperatures inside and outside the room, presence of toxic substances, and stuff like that.

In Balscomb's case, the one-inch thick round bulletproof translucent portlight in the door was to let people inside see if there were flames outside the door.

My other question is about ventilation and protection against toxic fumes being pumped into the room. The executive declines to answer that question, claiming it is one of the company's most closely guarded secrets, but he assures me that it is safe to use and also attached to an emergency battery-operated life support system with only 3" ducting that automatically kicks in whenever necessary.

He listens to my entire explanation of all the details of the Balscomb case and is confused as the rest of us. He has absolutely no idea of how anyone could have been seen inside that room and then escaped prior to the entry crew's opening of the door.

The most interesting thing I learn from my visit with him is the fact that there was a surveillance camera watching the hallway outside the Balscomb's safe-room. It is activated only when one of the panic buttons is pressed, but it still should show if anyone used the hallway to get away after the room was sealed off.

Using the executive's information as to where Balscomb's camera, videotape recorder and black box are hidden, I call Jack Bibberman and arrange for him to get Myra's permission to visit the scene and remove those items, promising to turn any new evidence we discover over to her, if and when she makes a formal case filing against anyone.

If for no other reason, the information about the camera and black box was worth the trip. The visit with my old friend in Pennsylvania was very nice, except for the interesting event that happened while we were eating in a small, allegedly Italian restaurant in Frenchtown, New Jersey. In between the soup and the main course, I heard a loud siren in the distance. A little while later the proprietor let us know that if we wanted to get the rest of our food we would have to come to the kitchen and pick it up ourselves. Our waiter was a volunteer fireman and the siren we heard wasn't a fire engine... it was the firehouse sending out a signal that all volunteers should report immediately. This is the only eating establishment I've ever been in where the most desirable table in the place is the one closest to the kitchen.

While driving my rented Cadillac back to the airport, a call comes in on my cell phone. It's Jack Bibberman letting me know that he retrieved the surveillance videotape and the 'black box' from the Balscomb house, and that the footage was very interesting... not for what was on it, but for what wasn't on it. Jack says he watched the tape for the entire six hours of its running time after it was automatically activated by a panic button being pressed. All he saw was the hallway, the witnesses, and the police and entry crew breaking in. Schwartzi was not seen leaving.

7

I'm getting quite familiar with 'square one' because I go back there to visit it so often. I keep thinking about that video all the way back to California. Jack says that the only sign of anyone leaving that safe-room was right at the beginning of the tape when for the first second or two the tape showed Marian's back as she walked down the hallway, away from Balscomb's room and out of camera view. This means that the panic button must have been pressed just after she left, and closed the regular door behind her. I tell Jack to give the new items to the kid. Let her do some of the work.

A panic button couldn't have been pressed before Marian left the room because the executive told me that the camera and doors are both activated at the same time the panic button is pressed. Because the buttons are all many feet from one of the doors, it's impossible for someone to press the button and then still get out and almost ten feet down the hallway before the doors slam shut.

Shortly after getting off of my return flight at LAX in California, I look around and appreciate being back in the land of make believe. From the moment my plane took off from here a few days ago, all during my visits to Mount Vernon New York and Buck's County Pennsylvania, I didn't see one attractive girl. Not one California sun-tanned blonde. I miss that type of scenery, and you never appreciate it more than when it's not available. Even Laverne will look pretty good tonight.

I can't eat this greasy French toast any more. I don't know how anyone can. From now on I'm going back to oatmeal, before my arteries get completely clogged up. The houseboat rocks a little, but this time it's not a dog-mail. It's Jack Bibberman.

"Hello Mister Sharp. Suzi said this is where I'd find you. She would have sent you a message, but for some reason the dog didn't want to deliver it here."

"Yeah, it must have been something he ate. What's up Jack?"

"Suzi's says that the attorney representing Jessie Balscomb sent over some written interrogatories that you guys are supposed to answer.

I thank Jack for the message and head back to the boat to do some legal research and preparation. When I call Myra to let her know that Morris Arthur's the guy who made an unsuccessful attempt to blame that fatal car accident on Suzi's mother and is now making a claim to defeat Suzi's creditor rights, she promises that unofficially I'll get the full cooperation of her office with my case. There's no sense asking her to try and look for a motive in the Schwartz hit-and-run matter, because anything hinting that Schwartz' death was not an accident would complicate her whole theory about Schwartz being Balscomb's shooter. I call Jack B. back and tell him to start looking into Schwartz' affairs. There might be something there we can use.

During this past week there have been a steady stream of visitors to our boat. I recognize some of them, but the others are all strangers. I guess the kid is trying to keep up her end of the bargain. She agreed to solve this locked room mystery to give me something to work with, and it looks she's really trying.

Even without knowing who her investigators are, I can tell by the checks being written from our account that they're all expert witnesses in the area of construction and engineering. There's also an 'optics' expert and some video technicians, as well as another round-trip first-class air ticket to Mount Vernon New York. She hasn't mentioned anything to me about my going back there, so maybe I guess she's planning on flying someone from Secure-Co out here.

Our attorney service messenger has been here several times to pick up paperwork, so maybe I'll be going to court soon. I certainly hope she plans on giving me a full report, because after being dead, sick, or broke, making a fool out of myself in court is my least favorite thing.

I can't take the suspense any more. I'm going over to the Santa Monica courthouse to take a look at the civil case file on the Balscomb matter to see what's going on. What I see in the file amazes me. The kid has bootstrapped her position as a creditor of the Schwartz estate to claim standing in an action of malicious prosecution, contending that the Balscomb estate has no case to begin with and that their wrongful death action is being done maliciously and only with intent to profit financially from the Schwartz estate.

She also contends that attorney Morris Arthur should be charged with knowledge of the malicious intent of his client, and that he should be joined as a party defendant in the her action. Demand is also made for a transcript of the trial to be paid for by the court and forwarded to the State Bar's Disciplinary Board for disbarment proceedings to be instituted against attorney Morris Arthur. I hope she never decides to go after me.

Her final demand is for huge punitive damages against the Balscomb plaintiffs and their attorney. The most amazing thing of all is that she's requesting all these things without asking for a trial. She expects it all to be awarded to her at a pretrial motion for Summary Judgment, the type of motion that's rarely granted. Of course everything is filed with my name as attorney of record. Nice. She's fired every piece of ammunition known to the legal community, and now she's hiding behind me in case anyone fires back.

I'm now heading back to the boat to research everything I can about Summary Judgments in the State of California, because knowledge about that subject may make the difference between my continuing as an attorney in this state or being laughed out of court and sued into bankruptcy. There's an old saying: when you shoot at a king, you can't afford to miss. With the papers the kid has already filed having my name appearing as attorney of record, she's taking one big shot. Not necessarily at a king, but at a fiendishly devious attorney. I hope she doesn't miss.

In California, our Rule of Court number 342 sets forth the requirements for bringing this type of motion. It also sets forth the documents that must be used to support all contentions made.

In essence, what it says to the judge is: "Your Honor, the Plaintiffs don't know what they're talking about. They have no case, so we want you to throw it out now and declare us the winner without even giving them a chance to waste the court's time with a trial."

When put in those words, it's easy to see why the courts are reluctant to grant motions of this sort. They don't like to see a person lose without having been given the chance to put up a fight, so if we bring this motion, the burden of proof is upon us to show the judge that we're right on point with every contention we make.

Once we take our best shot, the other side then gets a chance to show how wrong we are, and in this case I think they actually do have enough facts and law on their side to justify the judge in denying our motion and setting the matter for trial.

The big risk you take when bringing a motion like this is if you expect to have any kind of a chance of winning, you have to disclose everything you've got, On the other hand, when your opponents put on their opposition to your motion, you get a chance to see everything that they have.

A motion like this operates like a mini-trial in reverse. In a regular trial, the plaintiff puts on its case and then the defendant put its case. In a motion like this, the defendant gets to take the first shot. The court expects to all the same things you'd bring into a trial, so in effect, you're putting all your eggs into that one basket.

I can't remember ever seeing one of these motions granted, but I suppose in the stratified world of corporate litigation, some of them succeed. For the rest of us it's usually the actual trial where the battle takes place, and if the kid expects us to win a summary judgment, I hope she's ready to prove up the whole case... including a solution to our locked-room mystery.

From all that I've read, there seems to be a pattern with locked-room mysteries, and I think I have a possible theory about this one. I call Myra's office to let her in on my brainstorm.

"What is it Peter? Has Suzi solved the case yet?"

"You know, she's not the only person on this boat with a brain."

"Oh yeah, I forgot about the dog."

Her sarcasm doesn't' even slow me down. "Thanks, but I think I might have an answer. Have you considered suicide? Let's face it. There's no way anyone could have gotten in or out of that room once the steel doors slid down, so what if Balscomb did himself in? Have you done a psychological profile on him yet?"

"Nice try Petey, but you'd better leave the heavy brainwork for Suzi."

"Why? Tell me how you can rule suicide out."

"Okay, you asked for it. First of all, he was shot in the back of the head. Second of all, there were no powder burns, so even if he were a contortionist, he couldn't have shot himself from several feet away. Thirdly, the gun was found about ten feet away from him, and from the blood spatter pattern, our CSI unit estimates he was shot from that distance. Other than that, your theory is right on track. Any more questions?"

That was a let-down. Okay, so it wasn't suicide. There are other possibilities. I remember seeing an old movie where after the locked-room door was opened, it was the first person into the room who actually killed the drugged victim by secretly injecting him with a poison, while pretending to revive him.

I don't want to bother Myra again today with another theory, so I'll wait a day or so to work out the details before calling her.

In the past Suzi has managed to finagle her way into the courtroom on several occasions... once as my investigator, and once as one of Myra's subpoenaed witnesses for the prosecution. This time she'll have an absolute right to sit at the counsel table with me because she is the creditor plaintiff in her action to collect from Schwartz' estate. I hope she behaves herself while sitting there, because I know she has this strong urge to be a trial lawyer.

I think I've got a brilliant idea. This is a civil matter with no crimes involved, so Myra's being the District Attorney presents no conflict of interest if she sits at the counsel table with us. Maybe I can convince her to come in as my assistant legal guardian, to help comfort the kid and explain things about the case to her. If we can get a judge to believe that crap about the kid being a naïve innocent child, then we might have a chance. I'll have to talk that over with Myra. Sitting at the table between Myra and I should keep her in line during the hearing. Now all we have to do is convince her not to try and sneak the dog into court. She's done that before too, and the press loved it.

Ordinarily, Myra doesn't want anything to do with a case that I'm working on, but this one is all about her cute little friend Suzi, and our opponent is attorney Morris Arthur, who Myra would love to prosecute for something... anything.

According to the papers already filed with the court, the process has been set in motion. There are several rules about who should be notified and some definite time limits are required for the making of notice and filing of responses. From what I see in the file, it's going ahead right according to schedule, which means that the kid started it some time ago. As usual, she obviously knows some stuff about this case that I don't. She better clue me in pretty soon, because according to what I'm already starting to see on the news, this may turn into a media circus. It's got all the right elements: murder, mystery, rich people, a well-known magician, a locked room and a cute little girl. Who could ask for anything more?

The Motion for Summary Judgment hearing date is rapidly approaching. I've seen the witness list Suzi prepared for us, and it's got a lot of names I don't recognize. Unlike a criminal case where all witnesses are excluded until called to testify, this courtroom will be packed, and the witnesses will all be watching the whole show. Our list indicates that almost a half-dozen kids are included, so that means their parents will be there too. With a witness list this big and the press so interested, I wouldn't be surprised if this hearing is set for the largest courtroom... the one where Court TV's cameras are usually allowed.

I don't know why there are so many uniformed cops on our witness list, but who am I to ask? I'm only the attorney who's supposed to be in charge.

I don't know how I did it, but somehow I convinced Myra to join us at the counsel table. The judge made sure to let us know that because she's the District Attorney, she can't be present for any other purpose than to baby-sit with the kid. No questioning of witnesses or addressing the court on behalf of our case. Myra agreed with the judge's restrictions, and of course the kid is happy out of her mind that she'll be going to court with the closest thing she has to parents sitting with her at the counsel table.

The hearing date is rapidly approaching and I still haven't the slightest idea of what I'm going to say there. If the kid doesn't come through with something, I'm just going to have to look up at the judge and in front of the court, the cameras, Morris Arthur, and the press, stand up and say "never mind." I don't think my ego can handle a defeat like that, so I write out a simple message and wait for the mail-dog, who is temporarily busy with other important business.

This is the day of the month when Suzi stands on a milk-carton and uses her Flowbee-type of device to give the dog a haircut and hose-down/bath outside on the dock. After she finishes with the dog, several of our dock neighbors line up for a trim. Once the dog and our neighbors are replete in their sartorial splendor, I shake the biscuit box and put the message in his collar. It's a simple one that says "if you don't have something for me to win this motion with, I'm calling off the hearing and going to Maui for a week... on your dime."

Mentioning money always gets her attention, so in just a few minutes the panting messenger brings me her answer: "I'm working on it and waiting for results to come in."

That's not good enough for me. I have to try another theory with Myra.

"What is it Peter... another theory?"

"Don't be so closed-minded. I'll make it quick. Did your coroner fix the time of death? Because what if he was killed before the room was locked? I'm sure you guys have learned about the great deal of money involved in Balscomb's estate, and that's gotta give you some motivation to look at who's going to get it all. I hate to involve Marian, because she's a good friend, but all the information you have about what happened before the independent witnesses came to the house is from their statements. There's no outside corroboration, so why couldn't the two of them have been in on it together, to kill Balscomb, say that Schwartz was there, figure out some way to activate the steel doors and leave the dead body in there alone?"

The mere fact that she takes an extra few seconds to answer gives me the feeling that I might be on the right track.

"You know Peter, the thing that bothers me here is that you might be on to something, but for the fact that four independent witnesses gave statements to the fact that they saw the shadow of someone holding a gun pointed at the victim. If you have some explanation for

112

that, then we might have something to talk about. And as for time of death, the best we can do is narrow it down to the nearest hour or so, and because we were in that room within two hours, all we know for sure is that he was dead before we broke through the steel doors. So I guess it is possible that he was killed before the doors slammed shut, but unless you can tell me how someone killed him, pressed the panic button, got out before those steel doors came down, and then hypnotized the witnesses into believing they saw someone with a gun, then we're back at square one."

"So that's it? You've ruled them both out? What about motive? Did you see the victim's Will? He must have made one. Check with his lawyer."

"We did Peter. That's why we ruled out the maid. His will provided her with a salary of three thousand dollars a month plus room and board in his house for the rest of her life. Because that's exactly what she was getting while he was alive, the only possible motive she could have had for killing him was to save her from doing an extra load of laundry each week. That might have given me some motive while you and I were married, but cooler minds in our office decided it wasn't enough for Marian, so she's off the suspect list."

"Okay, I can live with that... she's a nice lady. What about the nephew? His uncle kicking off like that leaves him hundreds of millions. Did he have any gambling debts or other bad habits?"

"Yeah, we looked into that too. He doesn't drink, doesn't smoke, doesn't gamble, and doesn't have any unsavory friends. His uncle gave him whatever he wanted, whenever he asked for it. We even had our own doctor examine him at the scene and his pupils were still dilated from that trip to the eye doctor. He couldn't have hit the broad side of a barn if he tried. He wasn't the shooter."

"He could have hired someone to come in and do it for him"

"Oh, by the way Pete, his esteemed attorney Morris Arthur insisted that we give him a lie detector test and he passed with flying colors. You can draw a line through his name too."

"What about the maid? Did she take a poly too?"

"Mister Arthur doesn't represent her, so he had no standing to suggest that she take one too. And without any apparent motive, we didn't suggest that she go through it. Face it Pete, you're just not like one of your idols... and I think that Sherlock Holmes and Nero Wolf would have problems with this one too, so don't feel bad.

"Personally, I think that if anyone can do it, it's Suzi. She was right in the middle, being friendly with the Changs, who bought Balscomb's old house, and also taking those magic lessons from the other victim. We still haven't figured that homicide out yet. The only person connected to everyone involved in the case is Suzi, so maybe we should give her a chance to show us if her magic lessons can help out in the solving of this case. She's the closest thing to Eddie Poe that I've met in a long time, so maybe she can pull an 'Edgar' and drag your case up and out of the dumper."

There's no reason to burden Myra with the solution that my friend Stuart came up with, because he's a little far out when it comes to theorizing about criminal cases. In one of my weaker moments I allowed him to present his version of what took place in Balscomb's house, and the way Stuart has it figured out, a mysterious stranger disguised as Schwartz was admitted into the house by Jessie. When Marian left the safe room to fetch some refreshments, the stranger stepped out into the hallway, fired into the room killing Balscomb, and then tossed the weapon back into the room before the sound-activated doors slammed shut.

Being outside the room already, it was easy for the stranger to sneak out of a hallway window and escape.

As for the shadowy figure of a person holding a gun on the victim, Stuart says it might have been possible for a hologram to have been projected onto that translucent window. I think he's been watching too much sci-fi on television.

I have to admit that he covered all the bases with his theory. It might have been possible for someone outside the room to have done it, but how would that mysterious stranger have known to use the Schwartzi disguise to show up at the exact date and time that the magician was expected there?

Too many unanswered questions about this solution, but I'll file some parts of it away in the back of my mind. Maybe they'll come in handy to help me with the real solution.

I once read a book in which a famous fictional detective gave a lecture about locked-room mysteries and they all have one thing in common: once the solution is revealed, everyone is amazed at how simple it really was. I have a hunch we may all be trying too hard on this case.

8

Suzi's done some really nice work in the past, and I'm the first to admit that her computer skills have won some cases for us, but this time it's her own money and my reputation on the line and I'm afraid she's up against a mystery this time that's beyond her capabilities.

It might be possible to come up with some decent arguments on our behalf, but without a complete solution as to how Balscomb was killed and knowing 'whodunnit,' we really don't stand a chance to win this Motion. And if we can't win the Motion, we might as well fold our tent, because in this particular case, a lost Motion will mean an inevitable defeat at trial.

I try to use a back door approach to get some idea about what she's working on, but calls to Victor and Jack B. don't get me anywhere. They explain that this isn't a law firm matter because they were hired directly by Suzi. This also means that the result of their work is privileged. I have to agree with them and respect their professionalism. Damn. I feel helpless.

The hearing on our Summary Adjudication Motion is set for next week. Ordinarily I'd be busy preparing my argument, reviewing my research, interviewing my witnesses, and doing all the other things that lawyers usually do before going to battle. This time I'm not doing anything. There's nothing for me to do. We have no witnesses that can testify to anything that I think could help us, we have no evidence, and I have no legal points to rely on. Maybe the best thing for me to do is some psychological preparation for my inevitable complete public disgrace. The phone is ringing. It's Myra calling.

"Hey partner, what can I do for you today?"

"Don't you dare call me partner. I have nothing to do with your legal case. I'm only going to be sitting at that counsel table with you as an assistant babysitter. And the way this case looks, I'm even considering sending in a replacement for that."

"You mean your thinking of bailing on me?"

"Peter, you know I care for Suzi and want the best for her, but let's face it. I'm an elected official and you're my ex-husband. If I'm sitting at that table with you when it hits the fan, there's no way I can avoid getting some of it on me. I made a promise to both you and Suzi that I would be there, but right now I'm considering asking her to release me from the promise."

It's nice to know who your friends are when things get tough. I hope the kid realizes that she can count on me. I'm not going to let her know that Myra had thoughts of backing out.

I hear paws approaching. It's both of them. She's actually coming out here to talk to me, so I end my conversation with Myra. She understands the importance of a personal appearance by the kid and my wanting to get off the phone.

"Peter, I want you to know that I appreciate your willingness to handle this case for me. I don't know if I'll be able to hold up my end of the bargain. You said you'd do all the heavy lifting if I'd solve the mystery. I may be close, but time is running out for us. Maybe the information I'm waiting for will come in by tomorrow. If not, I apologize."

This is the first time I've ever seen a crack in her confidence. No matter how smart she might be, she's still a kid, and her enthusiasm in this case probably exceeded the reality of what she could actually accomplish. I'm pretty sure every parent experiences situations like this, so why should my raising her be any different? She honestly thought she could solve the case and I took a chance on her overly ambitious desire to win. The worst thing that can happen tomorrow is that we lose. Sure, I'll look bad as a professional, but that's part of the law business. Every time a case goes to court there's got to be a winner and a loser. I hope the public appreciates the fact that I stuck my neck out for a kid that I care for.

From news items that have been appearing, the public is aware that Suzi is the driving force behind our case, and that she's been doing most of the investigative work. I think it's time to call in some favors we may have coming, so while the kid works at her computer I'm going over to the Chinese restaurant for lunch today, and I intend to call in some markers.

The press has been following this case closely and they know the kid is trying to solve the Balscomb mystery. With Myra's help Suzi has gained free access to the crime scene and goes there every day to look at another part of the room, trying to answer questions she thought up the night before, and today is no different - and because the hearing is set for tomorrow, she'll probably be spending several hours there this afternoon. If she's getting close to a solution, whoever the guilty party is must make their move today or it will be too late.

My big yellow Hummer stands out like a sore thumb, so I told Jack Bibberman to go over on Pico Boulevard and get a car at 'rent-a-wreck.' He picked up a '99 Mazda, and we're now about a block behind Suzi's e-cart as she rides down the sidewalks toward the Peninsula.

When she gets to the corner of where Balscomb's house is, she makes her usual stop at the lemonade stand. After picking up two lemonades and giving one to the dog, one of the stand's operators hands her a note. Suzi reads the note and then looks down the street toward where a dark van is parked. She then hands a five-dollar-bill to the lemonade kid and leaving her e-cart and the dog behind, walks over to the van.

Approaching the van on the driver's side, Suzi doesn't see that on the passenger side, the large sliding door has opened and three guys with ski masks have jumped out. They run around the van, grab Suzi and toss her into the van. As they start to pull away, more squad cars then I've ever seen come out of nowhere and surround them. They must have been using binoculars for surveillance, because the only way they could've gotten there so fast is if they started to roll as soon as the masked guys jumped out of the van.

Jack B. takes her and the dog over to Myra's house for temporary safe keeping and to give me some time to cool off after seeing her pull off that stupid stunt. I thought she was smarter than that. How could she have allowed herself to get into that situation?

THE HEARING

Our usual procedure on days like this is to have Jack B. drive the Hummer and today is no exception. He picked up Myra at her office and is now waiting for me near the Marina entrance. As we drive down the street several reporters are following us. When Jack drops us off in front of the courthouse the press is waiting and they all seem to be shouting out only one question: "Where's Suzi?"

Myra ignores them completely. I make some feeble excuse like "she's not available this morning." The reporters don't know how to handle this. They seem to be afraid to ask anything about her health, so they just back off and inquire as to whether or not she'll be showing up later, to which my answer is "I hope so."

Using Myra's status as the District Attorney we access the private judge's entrance and hallway. When we walk into the courtroom through the judge's door, we see that the courtroom is packed.

Motions like this do not allow a jury, so the jury box is filled with reporters. I see that Court TV has some lights set up in the rear of the room, no doubt to be turned on just before the judge comes out.

The first row of seats is filled with the witnesses that Suzi has had subpoenaed, and I see that included on this list are Michelle Chang, her daughter Lotus, several kids that attended Lotus' 12th birthday party, the responding security officers, lead man from the safe-room company's entry crew, kids from the lemonade stand, and several others that I don't recall ever seeing before. The rear row near the door is filled with uniformed peace officers, many of whom I remember seeing at one time or another eating in Murray's Chinese restaurant.

We've been successful in keeping the attempted kidnapping of Suzi quiet, but I'm sure that word of yesterday's arrest has spread through the police grapevine. Looking over at opposing counsel's table I see that Morris Arthur is sitting there talking to both Jessie and Marian. When he finally looks up towards me I see a smug smirk of confidence on this face.

I'm not a violent person, and other than the two fights I was involved in while serving in the U.S. Army at Camp McCoy in Wisconsin, I've never attacked anyone... and those two battles were sanctioned,

125

because I stupidly forgot the Army's first rule: "never volunteer for anything." After discovering that the physical fitness program was actually a front to attract sparring partners for the Army's boxing team, I learned that it's not a good thing to hear only one bell in any boxing match you're in.

Looking at Morris Arthur, with his neatly trimmed salt-and-pepper goatee and blue dress shirt with the white collar, I feel like going over there and pounding his pomade-filled hair down into the counsel table. He even has the guts to walk over to our table. Myra refuses to look up at him. He notices that the seat between us where Suzi was to sit is now empty.

"Good afternoon Mister Sharp, Ms. Scot. I hope you won't mind too much losing today. I'd like to say it's nothing personal, but that wouldn't be true now, would it?"

I'm just sitting here, trying to ignore him and pretending to look through some papers in a folder. He continues.

"I see that your client isn't here today. I hope that won't affect your case in any way. Will you be asking for a continuance? I would strongly advise against it."

As he walks away from our table, Myra whispers in my ear. "I want him killed. Can you recommend anyone?"

Morris Arthur and I both notify the court clerk that we're ready to proceed and she buzzes the judge, who then puts on his robe and buzzes back to the clerk's desk, letting both her and the main bailiff know that the show is about to begin. The bailiff steps to the front of the room, stands in front of the bench and makes his announcement. "Remain seated and come to order. The Superior Court of the State of California is now in session, Honorable Ronald B. Axelrod presiding." As he says the word 'presiding,' the private entrance door behind the bench opens and the judge majestically enters and steps up, taking his seat on the raised judicial throne. He then picks up the file that has been placed in front of him and calls the case.

"Estate of Balscomb versus Estate of Schwartz. This Motion for Summary Judgment is being brought by a creditor of the Defendant Estate. Are both counsel ready to proceed?"

That's our cue. We're the moving party here, so I stand, state my name and who I represent for the record, and announce "ready to proceed, Your Honor."

This is followed by Morris Arthur doing the same on behalf of his client.

Seeing that Court TV's lights are on, the judge obviously feels he should make some sort of announcement concerning the nature of today's hearing.

"Counsel, Parties, interested observers, today's hearing for Summary Judgment, now called Summary Adjudication, is allowed by our Court Rules for the purpose of weeding out meritless or questionable claims before they get to trial. Sometimes they are used as a threat to encourage settlement, and I certainly hope that isn't the case here."

I notice that the judge is glaring down at me while he says that. He goes on.

"California has a policy of favoring trials on their merits, so I want the Parties here to realize that I agree with the State's policy and intend to be very critical of the moving Party."

He now looks directly at me while making his next statement. He wants me and the rest of the world watching that I'm going to have a tough time today.

"If you can't convince me that there's a very good reason why this case shouldn't go to trial, then you're surely going to lose this motion. Understand?"

I acknowledge my understanding. He has one last remark to make.

"The Court takes notice of the fact that sitting at the Moving Party's counsel table is Ms. Myra Scot, this County's elected District Attorney. While we are always pleased to have her present in our courtroom, for the record I would like to state that it has been stipulated that her appearance here today is in no way meant to be the County's endorsement of the Moving Party's motion. She is only here today to assist in the care of the Moving Party, who is a young child. By the way Mister Sharp, where is your client?"

"She's been unavoidably detained Your Honor, but as her legal guardian I am empowered to go ahead in her absence and offer her voluntary waiver of appearance at this time."

The judge looks down at me over his glasses and mutters a "very well." I have a suspicion that he may have been unofficially informed of the kidnapping attempt by someone. He looks down at me once again.

"Okay Mister Sharp, it's your turn. Please put on your case."

This is the moment I've been dreading. I have no case. This is a situation similar to the college student who has no idea what the answer to his essay question should be but still must start to write a few paragraphs, so he merely restates the question while trying to think of something else to fill up his answer booklet with. I stand up and start, hoping that what I say makes the slightest amount of sense.

"Your Honor, the Plaintiff's entire claim is based upon the assumption that the Defendant Schwartz was responsible for the death of Mister Balscomb. We have attached copies of the autopsy and investigation file from the scene of this alleged crime. There is not one piece of evidence that Mister Schwartz caused Mister Balscomb's death. The only way that Plaintiffs can succeed is if they present the trier of fact with a plausible way that Schwartz could have escaped from a locked sealed security room. A room that is bulletproof and soundproof, a room with no windows and with a steel sliding security door firmly down and locked in place.

"We ask the Court to take Judicial Notice of the fact that it took an entry crew over an hour to cut through the steel security door, at which time numerous sworn peace officers entered and searched the room, failing to find Mister Schwartz.

"It is merely a matter of logic, Your Honor: If Mister Schwartz was not in that room when Mister Balscomb perished, then he was not responsible for Balscomb's death."

I sit down and wait to see what happens next. The judge looks over to the other counsel table. "Mister Arthur, would you care to respond?"

Morris Arthur stands, buttons his suit coat and starts his soliloquy.

"Your Honor, Mister Sharp is obviously confused as to how the proceeding here functions. If he would have paid more attention to your very wise admonishment and explanation before starting, perhaps he would realize that we don't have to prove anything here today. The investigation record speaks for itself. Mister Schwartz was admitted to the Balscomb residence. He entered Mister Balscomb's secure area and Mister Balscomb was shot to death. It is not our responsibility at this hearing to solve the mystery of how he escaped... that is the job of the authorities in prosecuting Schwartz criminally. Due to the unfortunate fact that Mister Schwartz is also now deceased, there will be no criminal prosecution of him and we don't feel that the responsibility of establishing an escape route should fall upon us. We are not defending his actions here, we are merely seeking redress for them."

The judge thinks about this for a little while. I hear a lot of scribbling going on in the room. The reporters are keeping quite busy. The judge looks down at me.

"Mister Sharp, I agree with everything you said... but I also agree with what Mister Arthur said. It's true that if this were a criminal trial you'd have a pretty good chance of getting Mister Schwartz acquitted by causing some reasonable doubt, but this isn't a criminal trial, it's a civil motion hearing, and Mister Arthur has made an excellent point. I'm afraid that so far you haven't convinced me enough to shift the burden of proof and rebuttal over to the other side. At this point, I'm not feeling too good about your chances of success with this Motion. Did you pay attention to what I said at the beginning of this hearing? The only way I can hold in your favor is if no dispute exists as to either the material facts or the inferences to be drawn from disputed facts. In this case, there seems to be a great big disputed fact in your way, and that is the connection of Mister Schwartz to the death of Mister Balscomb. I'm afraid that unless you can go ahead and convince me that the facts are not disputed, then I'm going to have to deny your Motion. I also see by your witness list that you have subpoenaed well over a dozen witnesses to testify today, so I expect you to start calling them to the stand. It's bad enough for you to have taken up this court's time with your weak argument so far... I'd hate to find out that you've also wasted the time of all these innocent witnesses. Please go ahead with your case."

Myra has been concentrating on her footwear for the past twenty minutes. She doesn't even acknowledge my presence at the counsel table. A glance over to the other side reveals a terribly discouraging scene of attorney Morris Arthur smiling broadly, ignoring the seriousness of today's hearing and joking with his clients. He looks over toward me with one of those 'I've got you, you stupid idiot' looks. If I had a good hit man's name to refer to Myra, I might be tempted give it to her now.

I am now sitting here going through some papers in my briefcase, trying to make it look like as soon as the proper paperwork is located, I'll be continuing with the case. At the same time I'm looking down toward the floor, hoping to see a rip in the carpet that's big enough for me to drop down and crawl under. It's probably not there, because Myra's been looking for it since the hearing started, and if it was there, she'd already be in it.

The judge is starting to look impatient. Morris Arthur is beaming broadly, basking in his success. It's all over. This is the moment that every attorney dreads... our worst nightmare... being in court, losing terribly and having nothing to say. Please shoot me now.

Suddenly there's a commotion in the back of the courtroom. The doors are being held open by two uniformed cops and in struts none other than Suzi!

The press goes crazy. Some of them are running out into the hall, frantically dialing their cell phones. As Suzi walks to the front of the courtroom I see that Morris Arthur's expression is drastically changing, like he doesn't know how to react to this new development. His face goes from that pasted-on smile to terror, and then to confusion. He finally regains his composure. Suzi walks over to the other side's counsel table and glares at him. No one in the courtroom knows what she's doing over there, and that includes Myra and me. We're both sitting at our table in a state of shock. The courtroom is now completely silent and even the judge has been swept up by what's going on.

Suzi doesn't say a word, she just lifts up her arm, stands on her tiptoes, and slams down something onto Morris Arthur's counsel table, directly in front of Marian the housekeeper. Along with almost everyone else in the room, I stand up to get a better view of what it is she's brought with her and see that it's an hourglass with a post-it note attached to it.

With all the conversations going on in the courtroom that is still officially in session, I would expect the judge to be banging his gavel, but he's not. He's just sitting there like the rest of us, trying to figure out what's happening. Once again, the kid has succeeded in becoming the center of attraction and taking over complete control of the courtroom.

In a few minutes the commotion subsides, Suzi comes over to our table and hops up onto the empty seat reserved for her, complete with telephone directory for raised seating. Myra and I both look at her with questioning expressions. Out of the side of my eyes I notice that as Morris Arthur whispers something to his clients, he motions to the judge that he'll be back in just a minute, and he has started walking toward the rear exit of the courtroom. At that point, two uniformed police officers stop him from leaving the courtroom and instead direct him back to his seat at the counsel table. He does not look like a happy camper.

The judge looks down toward our counsel table.

"Well Mister Sharp, I'm glad to see that your client is here. Miss Braunstein, welcome to our court today."

She gives him one of those innocent little smiles as she nods in response. I don't know how she does it, but I swear she blushed a little. Myra also knows this is one of the kid's finest performances, so we exchange knowing glances because we see what the kid's doing. By playing the poor cute little frightened girl card, she's wrapping the entire courtroom around her finger. This is usually a sign that something bad is going to happen to someone soon... and I hope it's to people sitting at the other counsel table.

I look down at Suzi and the three of us have a little huddle.

"Suzi, are we ready to proceed? Did you solve it? Because if you would have seen what's been going on here for the past hour, you'd know that if you haven't got anything, we're dead in the water."

She looks up at me.

"Don't worry Peter. They're going to cave any minute now."

I can't believe this. Just because she walked over and put an hourglass on their table she thinks they're going to completely cave? No way. I'll bet anything that her confidence is a little out of whack here. My thoughts are interrupted by Morris Arthur as he stands up to speak."

"Your Honor, at the sole request of my clients, we have decided to no longer oppose Miss Braunstein's Motion for Summary Judgment. Also against my advice, my clients are dropping all claims they have against the estate of Sheldon Schwartz. This has been a tremendously strenuous experience for them and they want to put it behind them as soon as possible, so they can get on with their lives."

She did it. I don't know how she did it, but she did it. The reporters have a feeling that something happened, but they don't realize what the kid has accomplished. Whatever her placing of that hourglass on the table meant to them is still a mystery to me, but it must have told them that she solved it. And if she did solve it, she also knows who killed Balscomb. The bailiff walks up to the bench and hands the judge a note.

I feel a tug at my arm. The kid is pulling me down and telling me that she wants to testify. The judge is looking down at me and waiting for my response to Morris Arthur's abandoning his defense.

"Mister Sharp, I take it that you have no objection to Mister Arthur's removal of his objection to your motion. Is there anything you'd like to say?"

I look up at him with a pleading expression.

"Your Honor, if it pleases the Court, I'd like to have a moment to discuss this new turn of events with my client, to explain to her what happened."

Suzi glares and whispers angrily at me. "I know what happened. I made it happen."

"Yeah you made it happen all right, but Myra and I had to sit here twisting in the wind until you made your grand entrance, and that wasn't exactly fun for us. I've got to know what our plan is now, and if making you look like a dumb little kid is what it takes, then so be it. Now let's have it. What's our next move?"

"You have to put me on the stand to testify."

"How can I do that? The other side just caved. There's nothing to testify about."

"Yes there is Peter. The judge has discretion to award us legal fees, and that can be the excuse we use to call me to the witness stand."

"What's the big deal about attorney fees? You don't have a problem with that. Let's just get out of here while the getting's good. We've won. You've got to learn how to accept yes for an answer."

Her next remark catches Myra's ear.

"You really want to let two killers walk out of this courtroom?"

Myra can't control herself any longer.

"Suzi honey, what do you mean by that? Are there killers in this courtroom?"

It was bound to happen. The kid is giving Myra the eye-roll, indicating that the District Attorney, the top elected prosecutor of Los Angeles County doesn't get it either."

"Why do you think I subpoenaed all these witnesses? One of them killed Mister Schwartz and another helped in the conspiracy. Marian shot Mister Balscomb and Morris Arthur paid to have me kidnapped. Now please, tell the judge you want to call me to the witness stand."

"It'll never work. The judge won't go along with it."

"Yes he will... he's been informed what I'm going to do and he joined the program."

I now realize that it's happened again. I've lost control of this case, Myra, the

District Attorney of this County has no control, the judge probably doesn't know exactly what's going on, and the kid has completely taken over the case and the courtroom. I might as well play this thing out.

"Your Honor, if the court pleases, we would like to call our client Suzi Braunstein to the witness stand."

THE SOLUTION

My request causes Morris Arthur to pop out of his chair so fast that he looks like some pilot 'punching out' of a jet plane that's about to crash.

"Your Honor, we see absolutely no need to have this witness take the stand. The only purpose it could possibly serve is to determine responsibility for legal fees, and my client has instructed me to waive any objections to your awarding such costs and fees to them. Now that the matter of fees has been stipulated to, there is no need for the witness to testify."

We've got him on the run now and I notice that there is some perspiration on his forehead, and his client doesn't look too great either. It's definitely a high-stress time for the people across the room from us. No sense letting them get off too easy, so I take another shot.

"Your Honor, in certain instances the court has seen fit to impose punitive sanctions upon a Party, and we feel that this witness' testimony might shed some light upon whether or not that type of discretion should be exercised in this case."

Morris Arthur once again starts to argue. The judge cuts him short.

"Mister Arthur, I tend to agree with you, but this minor child has missed most of the hearing today and I think she deserves to feel like she's had her day in court. There's probably nothing she can say to create punitive damages where they don't exist, so just for the sake of making a child feel better, I'd like to give her a few minutes of this court's time."

The judge doesn't realize it, but he just signed a few death warrants. I've seen this kid perform in court before, and once she gets started, she doesn't stop until she draws blood. Following the judge's lead, I call her to the witness stand.

There are the usual oohs and aahs from the spectators as this adorable little girl walks up to the witness stand and waits there for a few seconds while the bailiff puts a telephone directory on the witness seat and then helps her up onto it.

I have no idea what she wants to say, so after she gets sworn in and the judge does his usual routine of asking a child witness whether or not they know the difference between telling the truth and telling lies, I try to structure the most general type of question possible. I want to give her an opportunity to say whatever she wants to say.

"Suzi, would you please tell the court in your own words, exactly what you feel the judge should know about this case?"

That should do it. She now has an opening wide enough to drive a Mack truck through. I sit down and relax because my job is over. I notice that Myra is reading a note that the kid slipped her. As she reads, she glances up, nods at the kid, and motions for a couple of uniforms to meet her in the hall. I have an idea that not everyone in the courtroom today will be sleeping in their own bed tonight. The kid starts out with her typical phony remark, designed to melt the judge and entire courtroom. She looks up at him with those googly eyes and a slight appreciate smile on her face.

"Thank you, Mister Judge."

That did it. She now owns him and every person in the room, especially the parents present with their kids. The judge has a look on his face like a proud Boy Scout who's just done his good deed for the day. The kid continues.

"First of all, I'd like to let everyone know that Mister Schwartz did not kill anyone. In fact, he was also murdered by the same people that killed Mister Balscomb."

Pandemonium in the courtroom. The judge is banging his gavel down so hard I'm afraid it's going to shatter like one of Sammy Sosa's bats, and become cork-filled shrapnel. The reporters are going nuts and at the same time three pairs of uniformed police come forward from the rear of the courtroom and arrest Marian and two of our male witnesses seated in the first row.

As the arrestees are dragged out, loudly protesting their complete lack of involvement in any crime, the judge looks down at Suzi.

"Young lady, you've caused quite a stir here today. I wonder if you'd care to enlighten us all as to what this is all about."

She sheepishly looks up at him.

"You mean here in court, with all these people?"

My God, what a ham! Not only did she take the whole place over, she's maneuvered the judge into giving her the opportunity she's always wanted... to be a television star on Court TV. The judge nods, signaling her to continue.

"First of all, Mister Schwartz was never in the Balscomb house on the day of the murders. Everyone was supposed to think that Marian the housekeeper called to invite him over, but she didn't. She made a phone call, but it wasn't to Mister Schwartz. The phone call was actually made to one of her accomplices... the one who was parked down the street from Mister Schwartz' house, ready to run him down later that afternoon as he was leaving his house for an appointment Marian had made for him earlier that week."

Morris Arthur butts in. There's a witness on the stand, so he feels he's got a right to interrupt her with questions. That's probably exactly what she wants.

"Wait a minute, miss. How do you know about phone calls made? We have sworn witness statements that she made that call. It was overheard by my client Jessie Balscomb and appears in his police statement."

Suzi's not going to give him an inch. She immediately responds.

"He may have heard a call being made, but he had no way of knowing what number was dialed. The police 'dumped' the phone records of the housekeeper and the residence phone and see that at the time she allegedly made that call to Mister Schwartz, she was really calling a cell phone that belongs to one of the people that District Attorney Myra just had arrested.

146

The car he used to hit Mister Schwartz is parked outside in the courthouse parking lot and the traffic division investigators have just verified that it was the car involved in the fatal accident."

Morris Arthur has just discovered that it's not a good idea to question her. He sits down and wipes some perspiration off of his forehead. Suzi continues.

"One of the other people arrested here today was another co-conspirator. He placed a time delay device in the panic button of Mister Balscomb's safe-room during what was supposed to have been a routine electrical service call to increase the house's wiring to accommodate more internet devices. The purpose of the delay device was to give someone inside the safe-room an extra ten seconds before the security doors slammed down and activated the surveillance camera."

Morris Arthur hasn't learned his lesson yet. Once again he stands up and makes a 'relevancy' objection.

I counter his objection on the ground that we will make an offer of proof, meaning that if her subsequent testimony doesn't prove to be relevant, it can be completely stricken from the record. The judge overrules Arthur's relevancy objection and signals Suzi to continue. He wants to hear the rest of her story as much as everyone else in this courtroom.

"With the help of the electrical delay device, the housekeeper was able to press the panic button, exit the room and get out of range of the automatic security cameras before the steel door slammed down and locked in place. The police never thought to inspect the panic buttons, so she had the next few days to have her electrician remove the delay device."

I can't resist the temptation. If it wasn't for the fact that Myra promised the judge that she wouldn't do any talking, she would probably be grilling Suzi now like a piece of toast. I have to ask a couple of questions, if for no other reason than my own curiosity. I also enjoy the positions we now occupy. For once she has to answer me, and can't just do an about-face and head for the foreward stateroom.

"Suzi, if Marian was able to leave the room, how did Mister Schwartz get out later?"

"Oh, that's easy. Mister Schwartz was never in the room. That's why the police didn't find him after they finally broke into the room."

She may have answered one question, but it only leads to more, in my mind.

"If Mister Schwartz was never in the room, who killed Mister Balscomb? And who was it that followed Jessie up the stairs to the safe-room? And what happened to whoever it was that went into the room?"

"Oh that's easy. When they first got home after Jessie's eye doctor appointment, Jessie was in the car napping for a few minutes while Marian carried the groceries in. That's when she followed Mister Balscomb into his room and shot him. She had to do it then, because with the steel doors up, Jessie would have heard the shot if he was in the house. She then closed the normal wood door to Mister Balscomb's room and went downstairs to fetch Jessie. Her whole plan was to have everything go down on the day of Jessie's annual eye doctor appointment.

"A little while later she led Jessie to believe that his uncle wanted to call Mister Schwartz to invite him over. Marian knew that Jessie's eyes were still dilated from his doctor's appointment, so she made the call to her co-conspirator from the hall outside Jessie's room, letting him listen in and believe that Mister Schwartz would be there in a little while.

"Then Marian went back into Mister Balscomb's room and put on her Great

Schwartzi disguise. She then called Jessie and asked him to put his hourglass on the hall table. Ordinarily the hourglass was on his dresser, but Marian purposely moved it when cleaning that morning, so that Jessie would have to go to the other side of his room to get it.

"When Jessie was turned around getting the hourglass, Marian slipped past his room, went downstairs and stepped outside the front door. She then rang the doorbell. Jessie had been instructed to go downstairs and let Mister Schwartz in, so still with dilated eyes, he opened the front door and thought he was letting Mister Schwartz in.

"The disguised Marian then followed Jessie up the stairs. When Jessie went into his room, Marian picked the hourglass up off the hall table, went into Mister Balscomb's room and in her own voice pretended to be welcoming Mister Schwartz. That's what Jessie heard from his room.

"Now that the scene was set, Marian got out of her Great Schwartzi costume, pressed the panic button and then exited the room, knowing she would have an extra few seconds to get out of camera range. She even stopped by Jessie's room to ask if he wanted any refreshments.

"That's how Mister Balscomb got killed and how Mister Schwartz's alleged escape from the room was pulled off."

I hate to do this, but a question is in order here, and if the kid doesn't have the right answer, her whole solution is in the dumper.

"One question Miss Braunstein. We know that the room was wired for sound, so that a gunshot would have activated the panic response. If the housekeeper shot Mister Balscomb, why weren't the doors closed at that time?"

Suzi glares down at me with the closest thing to a look of respect I've ever seen on her face. I think she realizes that I've just hit a weak spot in her theory. She takes a second before starting her answer.

"That was a big problem, but I finally figured it out. There had to be some tolerance level to the sound detector, so I had my investigators check the factory specifications and learned that a gun fired through a large pillow would be muffled enough to be beneath the level required to activate the panic devices. I knew that it would have to at least be a noise louder than a door being slammed, so we made some tests.

"Not being in a hurry because Jessie was still outside sleeping in the car, she

151

had plenty of time to get rid of the punctured pillow."

You can hear the proverbial pin drop in the courtroom. Even Morris Arthur is spellbound by her story. This time it's the judge who can't resist butting in with a question... and we now see that she's got him completely wrapped up too, because he refers to her on a first name basis.

"Suzi, I understand everything you said up to this point, but I still don't know how it was possible for the witnesses to have seen the shadow of who they thought was Mister Schwartz holding that gun on Mister Balscomb. Could you explain that for me please?"

Great question, and one that I was waiting to hear. Myra was too, because that and the other details the kid might now reveal will be the basis for her criminal prosecutions. The kid doesn't disappoint us.

"Oh yes, the shadow. Before the panic button was pressed, Marian stood up on a chair and opened up the portlight on the steel security door. This was done so that after the door slid down, people outside the room would be able to see the shadow inside the room.

"She then turned on Mister Balscomb's reading light and placed the hourglass in front of it. With the sand up in the top half of the glass, the reading light shone through the clear bottom half of the hourglass and made it act like a lens, throwing an image on the opposite wall. The regular reading light bulb was replaced with a special flickering bulb, so that the shadow would appear to be less than stationary.

"The shadow effect was accomplished by Marian painting a small outline onto the side of the clear hourglass bottom-half. She was very capable of this because she was an instructor in porcelain painting, and she had plenty of time to experiment with the proper proportions required.

"The witnesses were all able to see the shadow only until the sand came down into the bottom half of the hourglass, and then everything went dark. She rigged a small platform that the reading lamp was precariously perched on by propping it up with a piece of ice, knowing that after a certain period of time it would melt and the reading lamp would fall to the floor, breaking her special flicker bulb.

"No one noticed the tiny shadow figure painted on the hourglass, because when everyone went into the room, the painting was on the part of the glass that filled with sand, and the paint was the same color as the dark sand. In case anyone noticed, she even added a few other small painted figures, so that it would look like a design. By the time that the police got into the room, the melted ice's water spot had already dried.

"After the police were through with the crime scene, Marian removed the hourglass and no one noticed it was missing, but I didn't see it there when I visited the scene several days later – and it did appear in the police crime-scene photos, so I knew someone had taken it."

Wow. Over the years I've read a lot of locked-room mysteries, but one outdoes them all.

Before leaving the courtroom I address the judge and request that he modify his ruling so that all we are granted is Partial Summary Adjudication, which rules on the main issue point of dismissal, but leaves the issue of monetary damages for a future hearing. This will give us an opportunity to gather up all of our receipts and go for the maximum amount of reimbursement, including a reasonable hourly rate for the successful lawyer. The kid is especially pleased to hear that, because it means the other side will be stuck for my fee and all costs of the investigation, and if I know the way her brain works, we'll soon be filing an action against Morris Arthur and his client for the intentional tort of filing an unjustified lawsuit against our client.

Later that evening at dinner Myra has a few additional questions about motive and other loose ends she's going to have to tie up in order to get convictions. While sitting there in the restaurant we see Suzi's performance on Court TV being re-run on the evening news. Tonight it upstaged the Spanish TV soccer broadcast.

Many of the reporters follow us to the restaurant after court. They just want to sit around and listen to Suzi talk more about the case. I make sure to let them know that our dinner check is to be covered by their expense accounts. There are no objections, so I order a round of Patrón Margaritas, and the most expensive fish dinner on the menu. Chicken is out, because I don't see the owner's cat around anywhere.

I'm especially curious to know what Suzi knew and when she knew it, because I want to know whether or not to be mad at her for keeping me in suspense. From what she tells us, she knew that Schwartz never went to Balscomb's house because he didn't have a car, and the lemonade stand boys on the corner near Balscomb's house didn't see any cab drive down the street past them.

Michelle Chang was Suzi's porcelain-painting expert, and they succeeded in duplicating the shadow effort using hourglasses purchased locally that resembled the one in the crime-scene photos. The real hourglass wasn't found until later, when the police executed a search warrant for the rest of the house and discovered it hidden in Marian's room. It was really stupid of her to keep it, but once she painted that design on it, it became part of her art collection. After the case is included it will be a proud trophy in Michelle's collection.

Having been released from their respective confidentiality restrictions, Victor and Jack chime in with what they discovered. Victor saw Schwartz' body when he visited the morgue with Suzi, and made a GSR test of Schwartz' hands to see if there was any gun shot residue. He got a negative result. There wasn't any. This meant that Schwartz did not fire the murder weapon. His prints were on it because as part of her plan, Marian made sure that he held it during a prior visit to the house. She also made sure to use gloves when she fired it.

Jack had DNA tests performed and discovered that Jessie was not Balscomb's orphaned nephew... he was his son. And the mother was Marian, who Balscomb had an affair with many years ago. This started to highlight the motive portion of Myra's case. Jack also found out that Mister Balscomb had been so interested in magic over the past few years that he was considering changing his will and leaving everything he had to the American Museum of Magic – probably a recent idea he got from Schwartz, who mentioned that he intends to do the same. Marian overheard this while eavesdropping on Balscomb's conversations. She knew she had to do something to avoid this change, so she made plans with one of her porcelain-painting students who had confided in her that he started with that hobby while serving time in the penitentiary.

Through contacts with her ex-con student, she was able to retain the services of the hit-and-run driver that killed Schwartz, and the burglar alarm crook to install the panic button's delay device.

There are still a few questions remaining in my mind, but most of them can wait. "Suzi, why did it take you so long to put it together? From what you said, it looks like you had most of it from the start."

"I had to wait for the DNA results to come back. Motive was a weak point of the case. It also took a lot of time for Jack to track down every incoming and outgoing call from the Balscomb house and find out who the players were."

"Yes, but if you had the mystery solved, why didn't you let me know?"

"I had only part of it solved. Without the DNA results, Marian wouldn't have had a motive, and without a motive there was no one else to pin Balscomb's murder on. We also had to spend some time with the broken glass from that flicker bulb, and through her credit card receipts track down the hardware store where she bought it. If it didn't all come together, then we wouldn't have had anything, so I had to wait"

Myra still hasn't told me anything about the prosecution of those guys who grabbed Suzi, but I'm sure that'll come out later. I have a feeling that Morris Arthur was involved and acted on orders from Marian, who had heard of Suzi's mental prowess, and was worried that the kid's snooping around might give them some problems.

The dinner celebration is fun. We watch Suzi on television and eat ourselves into a coma, all paid for by the reporters. They're a little surprised when they find out that our dinner tab also includes the food and drinks all our guests had ordered, including Michelle Chang, Lotus, the lemonade stand kids and their parents, the entry crew, about seven cops, Jack B. and Stuart, who met us there and can eat like four people.

On the way back to our boat I can't help but let Suzi know how much of a risk we took by trying to defend Schwartz.

"You know, in the future, we should have more than just faith to go on before deciding to take on a complicated case. You honestly believed that your magic teacher didn't kill Balscomb, but as a result of just that hunch, we risked a lot of time, a substantial amount of money, and our reputations, all in the hope that he really wasn't involved in that murder."

She sits silently for a minute. I glance back at her in the rear view mirror and it looks like she's finally getting ready to let me in on something.

"You're right Peter, but I knew for a fact that he didn't do it."

"And when, pray tell, did that divine information come to you?"

"I was talking to Mister Schwartz on the telephone for almost an hour that day, at the exact time the murder was supposed to have taken place."

This is a shocker. It means she knew right from the beginning, but didn't tell me.

"You mean you knew all the time? Why didn't you say something to me? Why did you let me go on throughout the entire case not knowing that? What were you thinking?"

"Oh Peter, relax. It wouldn't have done any good. The only thing you would have then would be my word for it, and that wouldn't have helped any because I was not an independent witness. If I was to testify under oath about the phone call during the murder timeline, that might have been good enough to create reasonable doubt in the mind of at least one juror in a criminal trial, but we were going into civil court, and I didn't think that being a party to the action I could convince most of the jurors... I needed more.

"Stuart helped out a little too. He was on some stupid quest to find out about what goods and services he could get without paying sales tax, so I suggested he check out taxicab fares and directed him to whatever cab company Balscomb used to bring Mister Schwartz back and forth for the lessons. My lemonade friends told me that it was a green cab used every time, so we knew where to start.

"Stuart found the driver Balscomb always insisted on, and he verified the fact that Mister Schwartz didn't visit Balscomb's house that day too. That's why I had to wait until I had all my evidence together and had the solution. It wasn't just your reputation on the line you know, I have to maintain my credibility as a solver of complicated cases, especially when the press is so interested."

EPILOGUE

It looks like that law student magician was right after all. Now that the case is over, I see that it really was a simple solution. We totaled up all of our expenses, including my generous fee, and the court awarded it all to Suzi. She also got her fifty thousand dollars back from Schwartz' estate plus a little revenge by beating Morris Arthur, and her precious reputation as a child genius and courtroom Presario remains intact. She's pleased now.

But I'm not happy yet. I still have a couple of questions that remain unanswered. One of them is why a kid with her brains was stupid enough to believe that note the lemonade stand kid gave her, and walk over to that van. She didn't know I had the cops tailing her. That was a dumb and dangerous mistake to make, especially since she knew that Morris Arthur was our opponent, and how devious he can be.

My answer to that question comes out of nowhere when I hear a knock on our hull. Looking outside I see that it's Don Paige, our Internet guru and dock neighbor.

"Hi Don, what can I do for you?"

"Hello Peter. I was wondering if it was convenient for me to work on your Hummer for a while this afternoon."

"Sure Don. What would you like to do to it?"

He holds up a small device that's about the size of a deck of cards.

"I'd like to re-install your LoJack."

My LoJack? What is he talking about? I had that anti-theft device installed when I bought the car. If the car is stolen, the police computers send out a silent radio signal that activates the device's transmitter, which then sends out a signal that the police can then track to locate the car.

"Don, if it's the LoJack from my car, how come you happen to have it in your hand now?"

"Oh, I thought you knew about it. Suzi had me remove it when you started with that last case of yours... the one she solved. She wanted to keep it with her whenever she left the boat. If I didn't get a cell phone call from her every hour while she was gone, I was supposed to call the police and tell them to activate the unit. I guess she was worried that something would happen to her. You know how silly kids are some time."

163

Well, that answers another big question. The only remaining ones now are about the prosecution of those goons who grabbed her on the street and the collateral she was holding, because to the best of my knowledge it hasn't been returned to the estate yet.

I think Myra's in a better position to answer the prosecution question, so I call her office and get an answer that surprises me. From what she says, her office had to release the guys because Suzi refused to press charges.

"What? Refused to press charges? How can that be? You don't need her to press charges. Several teams of uniformed cops witnessed the whole thing. You've got their testimony... that should be good enough for you."

"You're right, but Suzi told us that if we try to bring them to court, she'll testify that it was all a game that she set up, and that there was no kidnapping involved. We held them for a couple of hours and released them to the INS. They were illegals and ultimately wound up getting sent back across the border to Mexico."

"Why would she do a thing like that?"

"I didn't know either, until she requested a chance to be alone with them in our interrogation room. I watched and listened from behind the one-way mirror. I couldn't make most of it out because she was speaking Spanish to them, but the gist of it was that she was only interested in nailing the person who hired them.

"She described Morris Arthur to them, trying to get them to incriminate him. Even I believed it when they pleaded that they didn't know that sleazeball Arthur, and were only doing it because some other Mexican fellow they didn't know paid them to grab her up to bring her to her own surprise birthday party. She must have believed them too, because they're now back in Mexico.

"I think she was going for a grand slam on this case... not only did she want to win the Motion, she wanted to solve the mystery and nail Morris Arthur, all at the same time. It would have really been spectacular if she succeeded, but she didn't."

Okay, I feel a little better now knowing that she didn't make a stupid mistake. No. On second thought, it was a stupid mistake. A little girl like her has no business pulling a stunt like that... using herself as bait for a kidnapping. It's going to take me a while to calm down about that, but I'm not going to forget about Morris Arthur. The next time I come across him, I intend to put him completely out of business.

One more question was answered when I bumped into Judge Axelrod's court bailiff a few days later. He handed me a small post-it note and said that he found it on the floor after we all left the courtroom that day of our Motion. Unfolding it, I see that it's addressed to Morris Arthur and I recognize the kid's handwriting. It says 'Mister Arthur. We have your Mexican friends. Please drop this case and we'll forget about your little plan.'

That little devil. She scared Arthur into thinking she had the goods on him for the kidnapping attempt and extorted a dismissal of the civil suit from him. Come to think of it, she probably only did it to put the fear of God into him for a few minutes, because once she started testifying he knew that the case was history. Technically he could never have her charged with extortion, because that would require him to come out of the closet and admit his participation in the attempted kidnapping. When Marian saw that the note was stuck onto Jessie's hourglass, she also realized that it was all over.

My only unanswered question now is about the collateral, so I use the maildog to request a brief meeting in the main saloon. They make their appearance and she is carrying a box filled with things I've never seen before.

"You mentioned that you held some collateral for that loan/investment you made to Schwartz. Now that the case is over and he's gone, can you tell me what it was? I haven't seen you return anything to the court, and I think you should take care of that before it comes back to bite us.

She puts the box down on the table and sets the sealing tape down next to it.

"Suzi, what is this box of stuff doing here on the boat? It doesn't look like ours."

"It's not ours. These are the personal effects of Mister Schwartz, and per his desire, they're all going to be donated to the American Museum of Magic, along with all the proceeds from the sale of the illusions we both designed. I'm packing them in this box and will tape it up in the morning, before UPS gets here to pick it up."

"The American Museum of Magic? I've never heard of it. Is it in California? I'd like to see that place"

"No, it's not around here, it's in Marshall, Michigan."

"Okay, then what about the collateral?"

She reaches into the box and removes a bound leather diary.

"This is it. It's a complete list of every trick and illusion he's ever done, and it reveals all the secrets. It's probably worth millions, or even priceless. With Balscomb's millions they would have been set for life, but she wanted something for her useless son Jessie to do, and he liked magic. That was her motivation for the lawsuit."

That's all the conversation I'm getting from her tonight. I saw her eyelids droop a couple of time already during this meeting, so I know that she's ready to hit the sack. She tosses the diary down onto the table, does her usual about-face, and leads the dog to the foreward stateroom, leaving me alone with all of Schwartz' personal effects.

For a while I sit back and contemplate the book of secrets, the magician's legacy that's lying on the table in front of me, easily within reach. At first there's an internal battle going on with my curiosity, because I'm a big magic fan... but my conscience ultimately wins out.

I lean forward, pick up the book and toss it into the museum's box. Once it lands with a thud inside the box I hear her foreward stateroom door close.

The Peter Sharp Legal Mystery Series

#1: *Single Jeopardy*

Attorney Peter Sharp has been wrongfully suspended from the practice of law and thrown out of the house by his soon-to-be ex-wife, a newly appointed deputy district attorney. As a result of the eviction, he's forced to live in their back yard on an old, poorly wired, 40-foot Chris Craft cabin cruiser he's restoring, that is in danger of burning up at any time.

To make matters worse, as the result of trying to help someone fill out some claim forms, he gets arrested for conspiracy to defraud an insurance company. His alleged co-conspirator, a man charged with murdering his own wife to be with a beautiful flight attendant, is about to discover that Peter is also sleeping with her while the man is out of town. As Peter fights to get his law license reinstated, he discovers the secrets behind two murders, a fatal plane crash, and who framed him with the State Bar - all with the help of his legal ward Suzi, an adorable, quiet (at least to Peter) ten-year-old Chinese girl and her huge Saint Bernard.

Peter also gets involved in matters concerning sexual harassment, vexatious litigation, double jeopardy, and a groundbreaking case of *Negligent Nymphomania.*

#2: *...By Reason of Sanity*

In his second Adventure, Attorney Peter Sharp gets retained to defend a man accused of capital murder. The only things making this case a little harder to defend than most others are that the client's acts were captured on videotape, he confessed to the police, and he wants to plead guilty. To make matters worse, the District Attorney's office has brought in a special prosecutor for the trial: Peter's ex-wife Myra.

While he's preparing for trial on the murder case, Peter is also hired to represent an insurance company, to defend it against a man who slipped and fell while inside a bank that was coincidentally robbed later that same day. Peter thinks the case would have died when the claimant was murdered, but at usual, he's wrong.

In this adventure, while Peter is involved representing Vinnie, the prolific, peeing pornographer, he also helps solve several bank robberies by catching the entire gang, and makes the acquaintance of a new friend who runs an autopsy store - all with the help of his legal ward, the adorable ten-year-old Suzi and her huge Saint Bernard.

3: *A Class Action*

In his third Adventure, Attorney Peter Sharp is retained to represent a man accused of murder, by the planting of bombs in vehicles. The client is also suspected of being part of a conspiracy to assassinate the President of the United States in an upcoming Fourth of July parade.

With the assistance of his legal ward Suzi, Peter cracks the case, identifies the real murderer, and at the same time solves the mystery of a dead body found in his friend Stuart's automobile trunk... all while falling for a lesbian lawyer, winning a Will contest, breaking up a stolen car ring 4,000 miles away, and battling with his ex-wife, who has been elected to the office of District Attorney.

In the adventure's finale, Suzi miraculously manages to get 'Bernie,' her huge Saint Bernard into a courtroom, where she makes her first official court appearance, holds her first press conference, and becomes a local television hero.

#4: *"Conspiracy of Innocence"*

Suzi once again saves Peter's case by finding the connection between two crimes that allegedly took place in different parts of the State, one of which Peter was arrested for. And once again, Peter falls for a woman who he thinks could really 'be the one' this time.

Peter's ex-wife Myra must make the decision as to whether or not she should resign from prosecution of a case in which she may have a conflict of interest – Peter's murder charge.

Everyone including Peter is sitting on the edge of their chairs as this double murder mystery comes to a shocking conclusion that involves a mafia hit man, revengeful drug dealers, a local police chief, and the ever-popular FBI.

#5: *...Until Proven Innocent*

Tony Edwards, A dock neighbor of Peter's, is charged with murder. Unfortunately, he is a suspended police officer with a known dislike for people who are the color of his alleged victim. He's also the subject of many citizen complaints for using excessive force in the minority community.

At Suzi's request, Tony has taught her how to help him re-load his target practice ammunition, also giving the little girl a basic course in ballistics.

When a local black movie producer who Tony was working for gets killed, Suzi and talks Peter into handling Tony's defense... which doesn't look too good because he was arrested at the scene of the murder with his gun still smoking.

Along the way, Peter once again gets involved with who he thinks might be 'Miss Right,' represents a 500-pound woman who is being discriminated against, uncovers a white supremist militant organization, and also stumbles onto a group of people who are pirating DVD copies of recently released major motion pictures.

Peter's ex-wife, District Attorney Myra Scot, makes a mistake when she subpoenas little Suzi to come and testify as a prosecution witness against the defendant, Suzi's friend Tony.

#6: *The Common Law*

Peter Sharp encounters a client with amnesia, who not only can't tell Peter what his own name is, but who also has absolutely no recollection of the crime he is charged with committing. In lieu of his memory, Peter's obtains video surveillance footage that establishes his client's guilt beyond a reasonable doubt.

The usual crew also gets involved, including Peter's close friend Stuart, Jack Bibberman the investigator, Laverne the 'amorous houseboat lady', and Stuart's employees Vinnie and Olive – who are having some disagreement as to whether or not they're legally married; and last but not least, little Suzi B. and her big Saint Bernard.

The law firm is still operating from their 50-foot Grand Banks trawler yacht in Marina del Rey, California... the vessel that Peter still doesn't know how to drive. As in past adventures, all involved continue to visit the local haunts.

One way or another each of Peter's cases winds up being a conflict with his ex-wife Myra, who is the county's chief prosecutor. He also may be more closely involved with FBI Special Agent in Charge Bob Snell than before, as they share a dangerous high-speed situation on a winding road.   Suzi's new friend Lotus and her mother also play an interesting part in this adventure as Peter finds that he is fighting a ring of credit-card fraud experts.

#7: *The Magician's Legacy*

Little Suzi has decided that she wants to study magic in this eighth legal adventure she participates in. Unfortunately, her teacher is the main suspect in what appears to be an 'impossible' crime... the shooting of a man in his completely locked 'safe room.'

In order for Suzi to clear her magic teacher of liability for this crime, she must convince Peter to handle the case, which he does under one condition: Suzi must help him by solving the mystery of this locked-room murder.

Her task is made difficult because all events took place in a secure 'panic room,' with steel doors in place, and no windows. Somehow, the alleged murderer is believed to have committed the crime and successfully escaped from a room that could only later be opened by a crew using blowtorches.

Suzi is especially motivated to solve this enigma when she learns that an attorney who she dislikes may be involved.

This is the most baffling locked-room murder mystery of the century.

#8: *The Reluctant Jurist*

There's a mini flu epidemic going around in Los Angeles and it has especially taken its toll among Superior Court Judges in Santa Monica, who all seem to have been infected at the same conference they attended.

Peter has been 'drafted' to fill in as a temporary judge for some civil matters, but winds up getting stuck hearing a big criminal trial involving a devious attorney as the defendant... the same attorney who Peter crossed swords with in a previous situation.

Suspense enters the picture when Peter's legal ward Suzi fails to appear as guest of honor at her own birthday party, and every local state and Federal peace officer in California wants to locate her.

This is the second adventure that Peter and Suzi B. have been involved where Suzi's Saint Bernard may be partly responsible for a successful conclusion.

#9: *The Final Case*

Suzi dislikes a certain devious attorney who Peter keeps coming up against. She feels that he has no business being licensed to practice law in the State of California.

When Peter's new romantic interest invites him to a cocktail party, Suzi and the other guests are shocked by a loud noise down the hall, coming from their host's study.

Other guests at the party include the chief of police, mayor, and district attorney, who unanimously conclude that the dead body they discover is the result of a suicide.

Even Suzi is inclined to go along with their conclusion… until she learns that the devious attorney she dislikes may be involved in handling some legal matters for the deceased.

Suzi won't let go of this one. Against everyone's advice, she keeps working to prove her suspicions about that devious attorney and his connections to what Suzi believes must have been murder.

The conclusion to this mystery is a complete surprise to everyone.

#10: *an Element of Peril*

In this tenth and newest Peter Sharp Legal Mystery, Peter faces a double task: defending a person who is charged with murder, and also trying to locate the missing victim, who was allegedly killed in a completely locked room.

Somewhere behind the tangled mess of a down-ward-spiraling celebrity starlet, a battling married couple, a missing currency trader and a dis-appearing corpse, attorney Peter Sharp and his legal ward Suzi must find where the truth lies.

As in the past, while Peter's client's trial nears, Suzi has failed to come up with any workable solution that can save Peter from certain defeat and humiliation in court.

#11: *a Good Alibi*

In Latin, the word "alibi" literally means "somewhere else," and to any person charged with a crime, it is an extremely valuable asset to have, because it can mean the difference between an acquittal and a conviction.

However, just having an alibi isn't enough: it has to stand up to scrutiny, because any good prosecutor knows that breaking an alibi and proving it was fraudulently concocted can lead a sure-thing conviction.

In this eleventh adventure of the Peter Sharp Legal Mysteries, Peter is forced into a role he never thought he'd be playing: that of a prosecutor. – and his main task is to break the airtight alibi that the defendant is using.

All twelve of the Peter Sharp Legal Mysteries are now available at bookstores and can easily be ordered online from Amazon.com.

To order at your local bookseller or online, simply provide the title's ISBN (International Standard Book Number), or insert it into Amazon's search block.

Single Jeopardy _____ ISBN 1-882629-19-1
...By Reason of Sanity _____ ISBN 1-882629-13-2
A Class Action _____ ISBN 1-882629-66-3
Conspiracy of Innocence ___ ISBN 1-882629-09-4
...Until Proven Innocent ___ ISBN 1-882629-51-5
The Common Law _____ ISBN 1-882629-39-6
The Magician's Legacy ____ ISBN 1-882629-15-9
The Reluctant Jurist _____ ISBN 1-882629-72-8
The Final Case _____ ISBN 1-882629-81-7
An Element of Peril_____ ISBN 1-882629-76-0
A Good Alibi_____ ISBN 1-882629-84-1
Legally Dead_____ ISBN 1-882629-75-2

Editor's note:

If you notice any typographical errors in the text of this book, please bring them to the attention of the author, who was the last person to sign off on the manuscript. We feel quite comfortable shifting the blame onto him for any errors he may have missed. He can be reached at: gene_grossman@yahoo.com

About the Author

Gene Grossman worked his way through high school, college, and law school as a shoe salesman, welder, process server, bail bondsman, tire changer, saloon piano player and 'extra,' appearing in seven motion pictures. He then spent 20 years as a trial lawyer, during which time he served as Dean of a small local law school, where he also taught several classes.

His film & video company produced over fifty special interest DVD titles on everything from boating, to bankruptcy. Now retired from the practice of law, Gene writes aboard his yacht in Marina del Rey, California, where he has just completed his twelfth. Peter Sharp Legal Mystery, **Legally Dead**

You can see pictures of Peter Sharp's boats, yellow Hummer, Suzi's e-cart, and Laverne's houseboat at

www.petersharpbooks.com

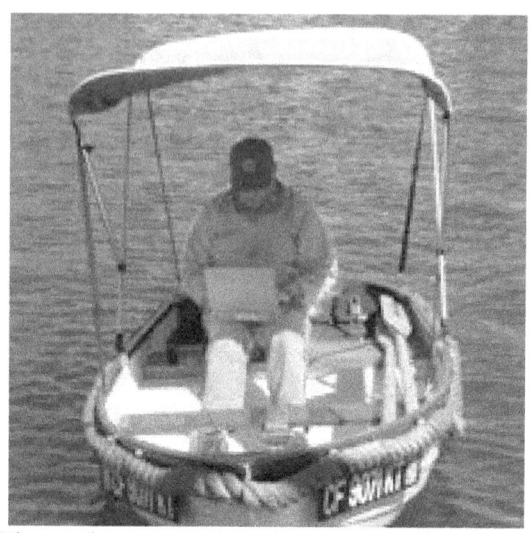

The author at work – always near the water.
In his dinghy, or in Avalon on Catalina Island.

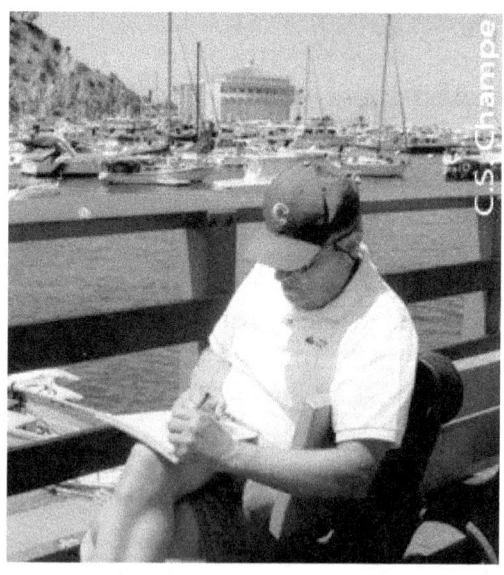

A note from the Peter Sharp Legal Mystery Series Creator

I first read the following story while a student in elementary school. It was one of the first books in my long passion of reading, and succeeded in getting me addicted to mysteries – first as a reader, and then as a writer.

Magic Lamp Press, the publisher of my book, has agreed to bend their rules to allow including my all-time favorite, along with the title you have just finished reading, in the hope that you will enjoy it as much as I did.

Another favorite of mine, Jacques Futrelle's Problem in Cell 13, is the first locked-room mystery I also read as a child, and that one inspired me to write this current book.

Cell 13 is included at the end of Number 9 in the Peter Sharp Legal Mystery Series, the Final Case, and I hope that you will read that one also and see what is considered to be one of the finest locked-room mysteries ever written.

Gene Grossman

THE GOLD-BUG
by Edgar Allan Poe (1843)

What ho! what ho! this fellow is dancing mad!

He hath been bitten by the Tarantula.

All in the Wrong.

MANY years ago, I contracted an intimacy with a Mr. William Legrand. He was of an ancient Huguenot family, and had once been wealthy; but a series of misfortunes had reduced him to want. To avoid the mortification consequent upon his disasters, he left New Orleans, the city of his forefathers, and took up his residence at Sullivan's Island, near Charleston, South Carolina.

This Island is a very singular one. It consists of little else than the sea sand, and is about three miles long. Its breadth at no point exceeds a quarter of a mile. It is separated from the main land by a scarcely perceptible creek, oozing its way through a wilderness of reeds and slime, a favorite resort of the marsh-hen. The vegetation, as might be supposed, is scant, or at least dwarfish. No trees of any magnitude are to be seen. Near the western extremity, where Fort Moultrie stands, and where are some miserable frame buildings, tenanted, during summer, by the fugitives from Charleston dust and fever, may be found, indeed, the bristly palmetto; but the whole island, with the exception of this western point, and a line of hard, white beach on the seacoast, is covered with a dense undergrowth of the sweet myrtle, so much prized by the horticulturists of England. The shrub here often attains the height of fifteen or twenty feet, and forms an almost impenetrable coppice, burthening the air with its fragrance.

In the inmost recesses of this coppice, not far from the eastern or more remote end of the island, Legrand had built himself a small hut, which he occupied when I first, by mere accident, made his acquaintance. This soon ripened into friendship --for there was much in the recluse to excite interest and esteem. I found him well educated, with unusual powers of mind, but infected with misanthropy, and subject to perverse moods of alternate enthusiasm and melancholy. He had with him many books, but rarely employed them. His chief amusements were gunning and fishing, or sauntering along the beach and through the myrtles, in quest of shells or entomological specimens;-his collection of the latter might have been envied by a Swammerdamm. In these excursions he was usually accompanied by an old negro, called Jupiter, who had been manumitted before the reverses of the family, but who could be induced, neither by threats nor by promises, to abandon what he considered his right of attendance upon the footsteps of his young "Massa Will." It is not improbable that the relatives of Legrand, conceiving him to be somewhat unsettled in intellect, had contrived to instil this obstinacy into Jupiter, with a view to the supervision and guardianship of the wanderer.

The winters in the latitude of Sullivan's Island are seldom very severe, and in the fall of the year it is a rare event indeed when a fire is considered necessary. About the middle of October, 18--, there occurred, however, a day of remarkable chilliness. Just before sunset I scrambled my way through the evergreens to the hut of my friend, whom I had not visited for several weeks --my residence being, at that time, in Charleston, a distance of nine my miles from the Island, while the facilities of passage and re-passage were very far behind those of the present day. Upon reaching the hut I rapped, as was my custom, and getting no reply, sought for the key where I knew it was secreted, unlocked the door and went in. A fine fire was blazing upon the hearth. It was a novelty, and by no means an ungrateful one. I threw off an overcoat, took an arm-chair by the crackling logs, and awaited patiently the arrival of my hosts.

Soon after dark they arrived, and gave me a most cordial welcome. Jupiter, grinning from ear to ear, bustled about to prepare some marsh-hens for supper. Legrand was in one of his fits --how else shall I term them? --of enthusiasm. He had found an unknown bivalve, forming a new genus, and, more than this, he had hunted down and secured, with Jupiter's assistance, a scarabaeus which he believed to be totally new, but in respect to which he wished to have my opinion on the morrow.

"And why not to-night?" I asked, rubbing my hands over the blaze, and wishing the whole tribe of scarabaei at the devil.

"Ah, if I had only known you were here!" said Legrand, "but it's so long since I saw you; and how could I foresee that you would pay me a visit this very night of all others? As I was coming home I met Lieutenant G--, from the fort, and, very foolishly, I lent him the bug; so it will be impossible for you to see it until morning. Stay here to-night, and I will send Jup down for it at sunrise. It is the loveliest thing in creation!"

"What? --sunrise?"

"Nonsense! no! --the bug. It is of a brilliant gold color --about the size of a large hickory-nut --with two jet black spots near one extremity of the back, and another, somewhat longer, at the other. The antennae are --"

"Dey aint no tin in him, Massa Will, I keep a tellin on you," here interrupted Jupiter; "de bug is a goole bug, solid, ebery bit of him, inside and all, sep him wing -- neber feel half so hebby a bug in my life."

"Well, suppose it is, Jup," replied Legrand, somewhat more earnestly, it seemed to me, than the case demanded, "is that any reason for your letting the birds burn? The color" --here he turned to me --"is really almost enough to warrant Jupiter's idea. You never saw a more brilliant metallic lustre than the scales emit --but of this you cannot judge till tomorrow. In the mean time I can give you some idea of the shape." Saying this, he seated himself at a small table, on which were a pen and ink, but no paper. He looked for some in a drawer, but found none.

"Never mind," said he at length, "this will answer"; and he drew from his waistcoat pocket a scrap of what I took to be very dirty foolscap, and made upon it a rough drawing with the pen. While he did this, I retained my seat by the fire, for I was still chilly. When the design was complete, he handed it to me without rising. As I received it, a loud growl was heard, succeeded by a scratching at the door. Jupiter opened it, and a large Newfoundland, belonging to Legrand, rushed in, leaped upon my shoulders, and loaded me with caresses; for I had shown him much attention during previous visits. When his gambols were over, I looked at the paper, and, to speak the truth, found myself not a little puzzled at what my friend had depicted.

"Well!" I said, after contemplating it for some minutes, "this is a strange scarabaeus, I must confess: new to me: never saw anything like it before --unless it was a skull, or a death's-head --which it more nearly resembles than anything else that has come under my observation."

"A death's-head!" echoed Legrand --"Oh --yes --well, it has something of that appearance upon paper, no doubt. The two upper black spots look like eyes, eh? and the longer one at the bottom like a mouth --and then the shape of the whole is oval."

"Perhaps so," said I; "but, Legrand, I fear you are no artist. I must wait until I see the beetle itself, if I am to form any idea of its personal appearance."

"Well, I don't know," said he, a little nettled, "I draw tolerably --should do it at least --have had good masters, and flatter myself that I am not quite a blockhead."

"But, my dear fellow, you are joking then," said I, "this is a very passable skull --indeed, I may say that it is a very excellent skull, according to the vulgar notions about such specimens of physiology --and your scarabaeus must be the queerest scarabaeus in the world if it resembles it. Why, we may get up a very thrilling bit of superstition upon this hint. I presume you will call the bug scarabaeus caput hominis, or something of that kind --there are many titles in the Natural Histories. But where are the antennae you spoke of?"

"The antennae!" said Legrand, who seemed to be getting unaccountably warm upon the subject; "I am sure you must see the antennae. I made them as distinct as they are in the original insect, and I presume that is sufficient."

"Well, well," I said, "perhaps you have --still I don't see them;" and I handed him the paper without additional remark, not wishing to ruffle his temper; but I was much surprised at the turn affairs had taken; his ill humor puzzled me --and, as for the drawing of the beetle, there were positively no antennae visible, and the whole did bear a very close resemblance to the ordinary cuts of a death's-head.

He received the paper very peevishly, and was about to crumple it, apparently to throw it in the fire, when a casual glance at the design seemed suddenly to rivet his attention. In an instant his face grew violently red --in another as excessively pale. For some minutes he continued to scrutinize the drawing minutely where he sat. At length he arose, took a candle from the table, and proceeded to seat himself upon a sea-chest in the farthest corner of the room. Here again he made an anxious examination of the paper; turning it in all directions. He said nothing, however, and his conduct greatly astonished me; yet I thought it prudent not to exacerbate the growing moodiness of his temper by any comment. Presently he took from his coat pocket a wallet, placed the paper carefully in it, and deposited both in a writing-desk, which he locked. He now grew more composed in his demeanor; but his original air of enthusiasm had quite disappeared. Yet he seemed not so much sulky as abstracted. As the evening wore away he became more and more absorbed in reverie, from which no sallies of mine could arouse him. It had been my to pass the night at the hut, as I had frequently done before, but, seeing my host in this mood, I deemed it proper to take leave. He did not press me to remain, but, as I departed, he shook my hand with even more than his usual cordiality.

It was about a month after this (and during the interval I had seen nothing of Legrand) when I received a visit, at Charleston, from his man, Jupiter. I had never seen the good old negro look so dispirited, and I feared that some serious disaster had befallen my friend.

"Well, Jup," said I, "what is the matter now? --how is your master?"

"Why, to speak de troof, massa, him not so berry well as mought be."

"Not well! I am truly sorry to hear it. What does he complain of?"

Dar! dat's it! --him neber plain of notin --but him berry sick for all dat."

"Very sick, Jupiter! --why didn't you say so at once? Is he confined to bed?"

"No, dat he ain't! --he ain't find nowhar --dat's just whar de shoe pinch --my mind is got to be berry hebby bout poor Massa Will."

"Jupiter, I should like to understand what it is you are talking about. You say your master is sick. Hasn't he told you what ails him?"

"Why, massa, taint worf while for to git mad bout de matter --Massa Will say noffin at all ain't de matter wid him --but den what make him go about looking dis here way, wid he head down and he soldiers up, and as white as a gose? And den he keep a syphon all de time --"

"Keeps a what, Jupiter?"

"Keeps a syphon wid de figgurs on de slate --de queerest figgurs I ebber did see. Ise gittin to be skeered, I tell you. Hab for to keep mighty tight eye pon him noovers. Todder day he gib me slip fore de sun up and was gone de whole ob de blessed day. I had a big stick ready cut for to gib him d--d good beating when he did come --but Ise sich a fool dat I hadn't de heart arter all --he look so berry poorly."

"Eh? --what? --ah yes! --upon the whole I think you had better not be too severe with the poor fellow --don't flog him, Jupiter --he can't very well stand it --but can you form no idea of what has occasioned this illness, or rather this change of conduct? Has anything unpleasant happened since I saw you?"

"No, massa, dey ain't bin noffin onpleasant since den --'t was fore den I'm feared --'t was de berry day you was dare."

"How? what do you mean?"

"Why, massa, I mean de bug --dare now."

"The what?"

"De bug --I'm berry sartain dat Massa Will bin bit somewhere bout de head by dat goole-bug."

"And what cause have you, Jupiter, for such a supposition?"

"Claws enoff, massa, and mouff too. I nabber did see sich a d--d bug --he kick and he bite ebery ting what cum near him. Massa Will cotch him fuss, but had for to let him go gin mighty quick, I tell you --den was de time he must ha got de bite. I didn't like de look ob de bug mouff, myself, no how, so I wouldn't take hold ob him wid my finger, but I cotch him wid a piece ob paper dat I found. I rap him up in de paper and stuff piece ob it in he mouff --dat was de way."

"And you think, then, that your master was really bitten by the beetle, and that the bite made him sick?"

"I don't tink noffin about it --I nose it. What make him dream bout de goole so much, if tain't cause he bit by de goole-bug? Ise heerd bout dem goole-bugs fore dis."

"But how do you know he dreams about gold?"

"How I know? why cause he talk about it in he sleep --dat's how I nose."

"Well, Jup, perhaps you are right; but to what fortunate circumstance am I to attribute the honor of a visit from you to-day?"

"What de matter, massa?"

"Did you bring any message from Mr. Legrand?"

"No, massa, I bring dis here pissel;" and here Jupiter handed me a note which ran thus:

My DEAR --

; Why have I not seen you for so long a time? I hope you have not been so foolish as to take offence at any little brusquerie of mine; but no, that is improbable.

; Since I saw you I have had great cause for anxiety. I have something to tell you, yet scarcely know how to tell it, or whether I should tell it at all.

; I have not been quite well for some days past, and poor old Jup annoys me, almost beyond endurance, by his well-meant attentions. Would you believe it? --he had prepared a huge stick, the other day, with which to chastise me for giving him the slip, and spending the day, solus, among the hills on the main land. I verily believe that my ill looks alone saved me a flogging.

; I have made no addition to my cabinet since we met.

; If you can, in any way, make it convenient, come over with Jupiter. Do come. I wish to see you tonight, upon business of importance. I assure you that it is of the highest importance.

Ever yours,   WILLIAM LEGRAND.

There was something in the tone of this note which gave me great uneasiness. Its whole style differed materially from that of Legrand. What could he be dreaming of? What new crotchet possessed his excitable brain? What "business of the highest importance" could he possibly have to transact? Jupiter's account of him boded no good. I dreaded lest the continued pressure of misfortune had, at length, fairly unsettled the reason of my friend. Without a moment's hesitation, therefore, I prepared to accompany the negro.

; Upon reaching the wharf, I noticed a scythe and three spades, all apparently new, lying in the bottom of the boat in which we were to embark.

"What is the meaning of all this, Jup?" I inquired.

"Him syfe, massa, and spade."

"Very true; but what are they doing here?"

"Him de syfe and de spade what Massa Will sis pon my buying for him in de town, and de debbil's own lot of money I had to gib for em."

But what, in the name of all that is mysterious, is your 'Massa Will' going to do with scythes and spades?"

"Dat's more dan I know, and debbil take me if I don't blieve 'tis more dan he know, too. But it's all cum ob de bug."

Finding that no satisfaction was to be obtained of Jupiter, whose whole intellect seemed to be absorbed by "de bug," I now stepped into the boat and made sail. With a fair and strong breeze we soon ran into the little cove to the northward of Fort Moultrie, and a walk of some two miles brought us to the hut. It was about three in the afternoon when we arrived. Legrand had been awaiting us in eager expectation. He grasped my hand with a nervous empressement which alarmed me and strengthened the suspicions already entertained. His countenance was pale even to ghastliness, and his deep-set eyes glared with unnatural lustre. After some inquiries respecting his health, I asked him, not knowing what better to say, if he had yet obtained the scarabaeus from Lieutenant G--.

"Oh, yes," he replied, coloring violently, "I got it from him the next morning. Nothing should tempt me to part with that scarabaeus. Do you know that Jupiter is quite right about it?"

"In what way?" I asked, with a sad foreboding at heart.

"In supposing it to be a bug of real gold." He said this with an air of profound seriousness, and I felt inexpressibly shocked.

"This bug is to make my fortune," he continued, with a triumphant smile, "to reinstate me in my family possessions. Is it any wonder, then, that I prize it? Since Fortune has thought fit to bestow it upon me, I have only to use it properly and I shall arrive at the gold of which it is the index. Jupiter, bring me that scarabaeus!"

"What! de bug, massa? I'd rudder not go fer trubble dat bug --you mus git him for your own self." Hereupon Legrand arose, with a grave and stately air, and brought me the beetle from a glass case in which it was enclosed. It was a beautiful scarabaeus, and, at that time, unknown to naturalists --of course a great prize in a scientific point of view. There were two round, black spots near one extremity of the back, and a long one near the other. The scales were exceedingly hard and glossy, with all the appearance of burnished gold. The weight of the insect was very remarkable, and, taking all things into consideration, I could hardly blame Jupiter for his opinion respecting it; but what to make of Legrand's agreement with that opinion, I could not, for the life of me, tell.

"I sent for you," said he, in a grandiloquent tone, when I had completed my examination of the beetle, "I sent for you, that I might have your counsel and assistance in furthering the views of Fate and of the bug"--

"My dear Legrand," I cried, interrupting him, "you are certainly unwell, and had better use some little precautions. You shall go to bed, and I will remain with you a few days, until you get over this. You are feverish and"--

"Feel my pulse," said he.

I felt it, and, to say the truth, found not the slightest indication of fever.

"But you may be ill and yet have no fever. Allow me this once to prescribe for you. In the first place, go to bed. In the next"--

"You are mistaken," he interposed, "I am as well as I can expect to be under the excitement which I suffer. If you really wish me well, you will relieve this excitement."

"And how is this to be done?"

"Very easily. Jupiter and myself are going upon an expedition into the hills, upon the main land, and, in this expedition, we shall need the aid of some person in whom we can confide. You are the only one we can trust. Whether we succeed or fail, the excitement which you now perceive in me will be equally allayed."

"I am anxious to oblige you in any way," I replied; "but do you mean to say that this infernal beetle has any connection with your expedition into the hills?"

"It has."

"Then, Legrand, I can become a party to no such absurd proceeding.

"I am sorry --very sorry --for we shall have to try it by ourselves."

"Try it by yourselves! The man is surely mad! --but stay! --how long do you propose to be absent?"

"Probably all night. We shall start immediately, and be back, at all events, by sunrise."

"And will you promise me, upon your honor, that when this freak of yours is over, and the bug business (good God!) settled to your satisfaction, you will then return home and follow my advice implicitly, as that of your physician?"

"Yes; I promise; and now let us be off, for we have no time to lose."

With a heavy heart I accompanied my friend. We started about four o'clock --Legrand, Jupiter, the dog, and myself. Jupiter had with him the scythe and spades --the whole of which he insisted upon carrying --more through fear, it seemed to me, of trusting either of the implements within reach of his master, than from any excess of industry or complaisance. His demeanor was dogged in the extreme, and "dat d--d bug" were the sole words which escaped his lips during the journey. For my own part, I had charge of a couple of dark lanterns, while Legrand contented himself with the scarabaeus, which he carried attached to the end of a bit of whip-cord; twirling it to and fro, with the air of a conjuror, as he went. When I observed this last, plain evidence of my friend's aberration of mind, I could scarcely refrain from tears. I thought it best, however, to humor his fancy, at least for the present, or until I could adopt some more energetic measures with a chance of success. In the mean time I endeavored, but all in vain, to sound him in regard to the object of the expedition. Having succeeded in inducing me to accompany him, he seemed unwilling to hold conversation upon any topic of minor importance, and to all my questions vouchsafed no other reply than "we shall see!"

We crossed the creek at the head of the island by means of a skiff, and, ascending the high grounds on the shore of the mainland, proceeded in a northwesterly direction, through a tract of country excessively wild and desolate, where no trace of a human footstep was to be seen. Legrand led the way with decision; pausing only for an instant, here and there, to consult what appeared to be certain landmarks of his own contrivance upon a former occasion.

In this manner we journeyed for about two hours, and the sun was just setting when we entered a region infinitely more dreary than any yet seen. It was a species of table land, near the summit of an almost inaccessible hill, densely wooded from base to pinnacle, and interspersed with huge crags that appeared to lie loosely upon the soil, and in many cases were prevented from precipitating themselves into the valleys below, merely by the support of the trees against which they reclined. Deep ravines, in various directions, gave an air of still sterner solemnity to the scene.

The natural platform to which we had clambered was thickly overgrown with brambles, through which we soon discovered that it would have been impossible to force our way but for the scythe; and Jupiter, by direction of his master, proceeded to clear for us a path to the foot of an enormously tall tulip-tree, which stood, with some eight or ten oaks, upon the level, and far surpassed them all, and all other trees which I had then ever seen, in the beauty of its foliage and form, in the wide spread of its branches, and in the general majesty of its appearance. When we reached this tree, Legrand turned to Jupiter, and asked him if he thought he could climb it. The old man seemed a little staggered by the question, and for some moments made no reply. At length he approached the huge trunk, walked slowly around it, and examined it with minute attention. When he had completed his scrutiny, he merely said,

"Yes, massa, Jup climb any tree he ebber see in he life."

"Then up with you as soon as possible, for it will soon be too dark to see what we are about."

"How far mus go up, massa?" inquired Jupiter.

"Get up the main trunk first, and then I will tell you which way to go --and here --stop! take this beetle with you."

"De bug, Massa Will! --de goole bug!" cried the negro, drawing back in dismay --"what for mus tote de bug way up de tree? --d--n if I do!"

"If you are afraid, Jup, a great big negro like you, to take hold of a harmless little dead beetle, why you can carry it up by this string --but, if you do not take it up with you in some way, I shall be under the necessity of breaking your head with this shovel."

"What de matter now, massa?" said Jup, evidently shamed into compliance; "always want for to raise fuss wid old nigger. Was only funnin' anyhow. Me feered de bug! what I keer for de bug?" Here he took cautiously hold of the extreme end of the string, and, maintaining the insect as far from his person as circumstances would permit, prepared to ascend the tree.

In youth, the tulip-tree, or Liriodendron Tulipiferum, the most magnificent of American foresters, has a trunk peculiarly smooth, and often rises to a great height without lateral branches; but, in its riper age, the bark becomes gnarled and uneven, while many short limbs make their appearance on the stem. Thus the difficulty of ascension, in the present case, lay more in semblance than in reality. Embracing the huge cylinder, as closely as possible, with his arms and knees, seizing with his hands some projections, and resting his naked toes upon others, Jupiter, after one or two narrow escapes from falling, at length wriggled himself into the first great fork, and seemed to consider the whole business as virtually accomplished. The risk of the achievement was, in fact, now over, although the climber was some sixty or seventy feet from the ground.

"Which way mus go now, Massa Will?" he asked.

Keep up the largest branch --the one on this side," said Legrand. The negro obeyed him promptly, and apparently with but little trouble; ascending higher and higher, until no glimpse of his squat figure could be obtained through the dense foliage which enveloped it. Presently his voice was heard in a sort of halloo.

"How much fudder is got for go?"

"How high up are you?" asked Legrand.

"Ebber so fur," replied the negro; "can see de sky fru de top ob de tree."

"Never mind the sky, but attend to what I say. Look down the trunk and count the limbs below you on this side. How many limbs have you passed?"

"One, two, tree, four, fibe --I done pass fibe big limb, massa, 'pon dis side."

"Then go one limb higher."

In a few minutes the voice was heard again, announcing that the seventh limb was attained.

"Now, Jup," cried Legrand, evidently much excited, "I want you to work your way out upon that limb as far as you can. If you see anything strange, let me know."

By this time what little doubt I might have entertained of my poor friend's insanity, was put finally at rest. I had no alternative but to conclude him stricken with lunacy, and I became seriously anxious about getting him home. While I was pondering upon what was best to be done, Jupiter's voice was again heard.

"Mos' feerd for to ventur 'pon dis limb berry far --'tis dead limb putty much all de way."

"Did you say it was a dead limb, Jupiter?" cried Legrand in a quavering voice.

"Yes, massa, him dead as de door-nail --done up for sartain --done departed dis here life."

"What in the name of heaven shall I do?" asked Legrand, seemingly in the greatest distress.

"Do!" said I, glad of an opportunity to interpose a word, "why come home and go to bed. Come now! --that's a fine fellow. It's getting late, and, besides, you remember your promise."

"Jupiter," cried he, without heeding me in the least, "do you hear me?"

"Yes, Massa Will, hear you ebber so plain."

"Try the wood well, then, with your knife, and see if you think it very rotten."

"Him rotten, massa, sure nuff," replied the negro in a few moments, "but not so berry rotten as mought be. Mought ventur out leetle way pon de limb by myself, dat's true."

"By yourself! --what do you mean?"

"Why I mean de bug. 'Tis berry hebby bug. Spose I drop him down fuss, and den de limb won't break wid just de weight ob one nigger."

"You infernal scoundrel!" cried Legrand, apparently much relieved, "what do you mean by telling me such nonsense as that? As sure as you let that beetle fall! -- I'll break your neck. Look here, Jupiter! do you hear me?"

"Yes, massa, needn't hollo at poor nigger dat style."

"Well! now listen! --if you will venture out on the limb as far as you think safe, and not let go the beetle, I'll make you a present of a silver dollar as soon as you get down."

"I'm gwine, Massa Will --deed I is," replied the negro very promptly --"mos out to the eend now."

"Out to the end!" here fairly screamed Legrand, "do you say you are out to the end of that limb?"

"Soon be to de eend, massa, --o-o-o-o-oh! Lor-gol-a-marcy! what is dis here pon de tree?"

"Well!" cried Legrand, highly delighted, "what is it?"

"Why taint noffin but a skull --somebody bin lef him head up de tree, and de crows done gobble ebery bit ob de meat off."

"A skull, you say! --very well! --how is it fastened to the limb? --what holds it on?"

"Sure nuff, massa; mus look. Why dis berry curous sarcumstance, pon my word --dare's a great big nail in de skull, what fastens ob it on to de tree."

"Well now, Jupiter, do exactly as I tell you --do you hear?"

"Yes, massa."

"Pay attention, then! --find the left eye of the skull."

"Hum! hoo! dat's good! why dar ain't no eye lef' at all."

"Curse your stupidity! do you know your right hand from your left?"

"Yes, I nose dat --nose all bout dat --'tis my left hand what I chops de wood wid."

"To be sure! you are left-handed; and your left eye is on the same side as your left hand. Now, I suppose, you can find the left eye of the skull, or the place where the left eye has been. Have you found it?"

Here was a long pause. At length the negro asked,

"Is de lef' eye of de skull pon de same side as de lef' hand of de skull, too? --cause de skull ain't got not a bit ob a hand at all --nebber mind! I got de lef' eye now --here de lef' eye! what mus do wid it?"

"Let the beetle drop through it, as far as the string will reach --but be careful and not let go your hold of the string."

"All dat done, Massa Will; mighty easy ting for to put de bug fru de hole --look out for him dar below?"

During this colloquy no portion of Jupiter's person could be seen; but the beetle, which he had suffered to descend, was now visible at the end of the string, and glistened, like a globe of burnished gold, in the last rays of the setting sun, some of which still faintly illumined the eminence upon which we stood. The scarabaeus hung quite clear of any branches, and, if allowed to fall, would have fallen at our feet. Legrand immediately took the scythe, and cleared with it a circular space, three or four yards in diameter, just beneath the insect, and, having accomplished this, ordered Jupiter to let go the string and come down from the tree.

Driving a peg, with great nicety, into the ground, at the precise spot where the beetle fell, my friend now produced from his pocket a tape-measure. Fastening one end of this at that point of the trunk of the tree which was nearest the peg, he unrolled it till it reached the peg, and thence farther unrolled it, in the direction already established by the two points of the tree and the peg, for the distance of fifty feet --Jupiter clearing away the brambles with the scythe. At the spot thus attained a second peg was driven, and about this, as a centre, a rude circle, about four feet in diameter, described. Taking now a spade himself, and giving one to Jupiter and one to me, Legrand begged us to set about one to digging as quickly as possible.

To speak the truth, I had no especial relish for such amusement at any time, and, at that particular moment, would most willingly have declined it; for the night was coming on, and I felt much fatigued with the exercise already taken; but I saw no mode of escape, and was fearful of disturbing my poor friend's equanimity by a refusal. Could I have depended, indeed, upon Jupiter's aid, I would have had no hesitation in attempting to get the lunatic home by force; but I was too well assured of the old negro's disposition, to hope that he would assist me, under any circumstances, in a personal contest with his master. I made no doubt that the latter had been infected with some of the innumerable Southern superstitions about money buried, and that his phantasy had received confirmation by the finding of the scarabaeus, or, perhaps, by Jupiter's obstinacy in maintaining it to be "a bug of real gold." A mind disposed to lunacy would readily be led away by such suggestions --especially if chiming in with favorite preconceived ideas --and then I called to mind the poor fellow's speech about the beetle's being "the index of his fortune." Upon the whole, I was sadly vexed and puzzled, but, at length, I concluded to make a virtue of necessity --to dig with a good will, and thus the sooner to convince the visionary, by ocular demonstration, of the fallacy of the opinions he entertained.

The lanterns having been lit, we all fell to work with a zeal worthy a more rational cause; and, as the glare fell upon our persons and implements, I could not help thinking how picturesque a group we composed, and how strange and suspicious our labors must have appeared to any interloper who, by chance, might have stumbled upon our whereabouts.

We dug very steadily for two hours. Little was said; and our chief embarrassment lay in the yelpings of the dog, who took exceeding interest in our proceedings. He, at length, became so obstreperous that we grew fearful of his giving the alarm to some stragglers in the vicinity; --or, rather, this was the apprehension of Legrand; --for myself, I should have rejoiced at any interruption which might have enabled me to get the wanderer home. The noise was, at length, very effectually silenced by Jupiter, who, getting out of the hole with a dogged air of deliberation, tied the brute's mouth up with one of his suspenders, and then returned, with a grave chuckle, to his task.

When the time mentioned had expired, we had reached a depth of five feet, and yet no signs of any treasure became manifest. A general pause ensued, and I began to hope that the farce was at an end. Legrand, however, although evidently much disconcerted, wiped his brow thoughtfully and recommenced. We had excavated the entire circle of four feet diameter, and now we slightly enlarged the limit, and went to the farther depth of two feet. Still nothing appeared. The gold-seeker, whom I sincerely pitied, at length clambered from the pit, with the bitterest disappointment imprinted upon every feature, and proceeded, slowly and reluctantly, to put on his coat, which he had thrown off at the beginning of his labor. In the mean time I made no remark. Jupiter, at a signal from his master, began to gather up his tools. This done, and the dog having been unmuzzled, we turned in profound silence towards home.

We had taken, perhaps, a dozen steps in this direction, when, with a loud oath, Legrand strode up to Jupiter, and seized him by the collar. The astonished negro opened his eyes and mouth to the fullest extent, let fall the spades, and fell upon his knees.

"You scoundrel," said Legrand, hissing out the syllables from between his clenched teeth --"you infernal black villain! --speak, I tell you! --answer me this instant, without prevarication! which --which is your left eye?"

"Oh, my golly, Massa Will! ain't dis here my lef' eye for sartain?" roared the terrified Jupiter, placing his hand upon his right organ of vision, and holding it there with a desperate pertinacity, as if in immediate dread of his master's attempt at a gouge.

"I thought so! --I knew it! --hurrah!" vociferated Legrand, letting the negro go, and executing a series

212

of curvets and caracols, much to the astonishment of his valet, who, arising from his knees, looked, mutely, from his master to myself, and then from myself to his master.

"Come! we must go back," said the latter, "the game's not up yet;" and he again led the way to the tulip-tree.

"Jupiter," said he, when we reached its foot, come here! was the skull nailed to the limb with the face outward, or with the face to the limb?"

"De face was out, massa, so dat de crows could get at de eyes good, widout any trouble."

"Well, then, was it this eye or that through which you let the beetle fall?" --here Legrand touched each of Jupiter's eyes.

"'Twas dis eye, massa --de lef' eye --jis as you tell me," and here it was his right eye that the negro indicated.

"That will do --we must try it again."

Here my friend, about whose madness I now saw, or fancied that I saw, certain indications of method, removed the peg which marked the spot where the beetle fell, to a spot about three inches to the westward of its former position. Taking, now, the tape-measure from the nearest point of the trunk to the peg, as before, and continuing the extension in a straight line to the distance of fifty feet, a spot was indicated, removed, by several yards, from the point at which we had been digging.

Around the new position a circle, somewhat larger than in the former instance, was now described, and we again set to work with the spades. I was dreadfully weary, but, scarcely understanding what had occasioned the change in my thoughts, I felt no longer any great aversion from the labor imposed. I had become most unaccountably interested --nay, even excited. Perhaps there was something, amid all the extravagant demeanor of Legrand --some air of forethought, or of deliberation, which impressed me. I dug eagerly, and now and then caught myself actually looking, with something that very much resembled expectation, for the fancied treasure, the vision of which had demented my unfortunate companion. At a period when such vagaries of thought most fully possessed me, and when we had been at work perhaps an hour and a half, we were again interrupted by the violent howlings of the dog. His uneasiness, in the first instance, had been, evidently, but the result of playfulness or caprice, but he now assumed a bitter and serious tone. Upon Jupiter's again attempting to muzzle him, he made furious resistance, and, leaping into the hole, tore up the mould frantically with his claws. In a few seconds he had uncovered a mass of human bones, forming two complete skeletons, intermingled with several buttons of metal, and what appeared to be the dust of decayed woollen. One or two strokes of a spade upturned the blade of a large Spanish knife, and, as we dug farther, three or four loose pieces of gold and silver coin came to light.

At sight of these the joy of Jupiter could scarcely be restrained, but the countenance of his master wore an air of extreme disappointment. He urged us, however, to continue our exertions, and the words were hardly uttered when I stumbled and fell forward, having caught the toe of my boot in a large ring of iron that lay half buried in the loose earth.

We now worked in earnest, and never did I pass ten minutes of more intense excitement. During this interval we had fairly unearthed an oblong chest of wood, which, from its perfect preservation, and wonderful hardness, had plainly been subjected to some mineralizing process --perhaps that of the Bi-chloride of Mercury. This box was three feet and a half long, three feet broad, and two and a half feet deep. It was firmly secured by bands of wrought iron, riveted, and forming a kind of trellis-work over the whole. On each side of the chest, near the top, were three rings of iron --six in all --by means of which a firm hold could be obtained by six persons. Our utmost united endeavors served only to disturb the coffer very slightly in its bed. We at once saw the impossibility of removing so great a weight. Luckily, the sole fastenings of the lid consisted of two sliding bolts. These we drew back --trembling and panting with anxiety. In an instant, a treasure of incalculable value lay gleaming before us. As the rays of the lanterns fell within the pit, there flashed upwards, from a confused heap of gold and of jewels, a glow and a glare that absolutely dazzled our eyes.

I shall not pretend to describe the feelings with which I gazed. Amazement was, of course, predominant. Legrand appeared exhausted with excitement, and spoke very few words. Jupiter's countenance wore, for some minutes, as deadly a pallor as it is possible, in the nature of things, for any negro's visage to assume. He seemed stupefied --thunder-stricken. Presently he fell upon his knees in the pit, and, burying his naked arms up to the elbows in gold, let them there remain, as if enjoying the luxury of a bath. At length, with a deep sigh, he exclaimed, as if in a soliloquy.

"And dis all cum ob de goole-bug! de putty goole-bug! de poor little goole-bug, what I boosed in dat sabage kind ob style! Ain't you shamed ob yourself, nigger? --answer me dat!"

It became necessary, at last, that I should arouse both master and valet to the expediency of removing the treasure. It was growing late, and it behooved us to make exertion, that we might get every thing housed before daylight. It was difficult to say what should be done; and much time was spent in deliberation --so confused were the ideas of all. We, finally, lightened the box by removing two thirds of its contents, when we were enabled, with some trouble, to raise it from the hole. The articles taken out were deposited among the brambles, and the dog left to guard them, with strict orders from Jupiter neither, upon any pretence, to stir from the spot, nor to open his mouth until our return. We then hurriedly made for home with the chest; reaching the hut in safety, but after excessive toil, at one o'clock in the morning. Worn out as we were, it was not in human nature to do more just then. We rested until two, and had supper; starting for the hills immediately afterwards, armed with three stout sacks, which, by good luck, were upon the premises. A little before four we arrived at the pit, divided the remainder of the booty, as equally as might be, among us, and, leaving the holes unfilled, again set out for the hut, at which, for the second time, we deposited our golden burthens, just as the first streaks of the dawn gleamed from over the tree-tops in the East.

We were now thoroughly broken down; but the intense excitement of the time denied us repose. After an unquiet slumber of some three or four hours' duration, we arose, as if by preconcert, to make examination of our treasure.

The chest had been full to the brim, and we spent the whole day, and the greater part of the next night, in a scrutiny of its contents. There had been nothing like order or arrangement. Every thing had been heaped in promiscuously. Having assorted all with care, we found ourselves possessed of even vaster wealth than we had at first supposed. In coin there was rather more than four hundred and fifty thousand dollars --

estimating the value of the pieces, as accurately as we could, by the tables of the period. There was not a particle of silver. All was gold of antique date and of great variety --French, Spanish, and German money, with a few English guineas, and some counters, of which we had never seen specimens before. There were several very large and heavy coins, so worn that we could make nothing of their inscriptions. There was no American money. The value of the jewels we found more difficulty in estimating. There were diamonds --some of them exceedingly large and fine --a hundred and ten in all, and not one of them small; eighteen rubies of remarkable brilliancy; --three hundred and ten emeralds, all very beautiful; and twenty-one sapphires, with an opal. These stones had all been broken from their settings and thrown loose in the chest. The settings themselves, which we picked out from among the other gold, appeared to have been beaten up with hammers, as if to prevent identification. Besides all this, there was a vast quantity of solid gold ornaments; --nearly two hundred massive finger and ear rings; --rich chains -- thirty of these, if I remember; --eighty-three very large and heavy crucifixes; --five gold censers of great value; --a prodigious golden punch-bowl, ornamented with richly chased vine-leaves and Bacchanalian figures; with two sword-handles exquisitely embossed, and many other smaller articles which I cannot recollect. The weight of these valuables exceeded three hundred and fifty pounds avoirdupois; and in this estimate I have not included one hundred and ninety-seven superb gold watches;

three of the number being worth each five hundred dollars, if one. Many of them were very old, and as time keepers valueless; the works having suffered, more or less, from corrosion --but all were richly jewelled and in cases of great worth. We estimated the entire contents of the chest, that night, at a million and a half of dollars; and, upon the subsequent disposal of the trinkets and jewels (a few being retained for our own use), it was found that we had greatly undervalued the treasure.

When, at length, we had concluded our examination, and the intense excitement of the time had, in some measure, subsided, Legrand, who saw that I was dying with impatience for a solution of this most extraordinary riddle, entered into a full detail of all the circumstances connected with it.

"You remember," said he, "the night when I handed you the rough sketch I had made of the scarabaeus. You recollect also, that I became quite vexed at you for insisting that my drawing resembled a death's-head. When you first made this assertion I thought you were jesting; but afterwards I called to mind the peculiar spots on the back of the insect, and admitted to myself that your remark had some little foundation in fact. Still, the sneer at my graphic powers irritated me --for I am considered a good artist --and, therefore, when you handed me the scrap of parchment, I was about to crumple it up and throw it angrily into the fire."

"The scrap of paper, you mean," said I.

"No; it had much of the appearance of paper, and at first I supposed it to be such, but when I came to draw upon it, I discovered it, at once, to be a piece of very thin parchment. It was quite dirty, you remember. Well, as I was in the very act of crumpling it up, my glance fell upon the sketch at which you had been looking, and you may imagine my astonishment when I perceived, in fact, the figure of a death's-head just where, it seemed to me, I had made the drawing of the beetle. For a moment I was too much amazed to think with accuracy. I knew that my design was very different in detail from this -- although there was a certain similarity in general outline. Presently I took a candle, and seating myself at the other end of the room, proceeded to scrutinize the parchment more closely. Upon turning it over, I saw my own sketch upon the reverse, just as I had made it. My first idea, now, was mere surprise at the really remarkable similarity of outline --at the singular coincidence involved in the fact, that unknown to me, there should have been a skull upon the other side of the parchment, immediately beneath my figure of the scarabaeus and that this skull, not only in outline, but in size, should so closely resemble my drawing. I say the singularity of this coincidence absolutely stupefied me for a time. This is the usual effect of such coincidences. The mind struggles to establish a connection --a sequence of cause and effect --and, being unable to do so, suffers a species of temporary paralysis. But, when I recovered from this stupor, there dawned upon me gradually a conviction which startled me even far more than the coincidence. I began distinctly, positively, to remember that there had been no drawing on the parchment when I made my sketch of the scarabaeus. I became perfectly certain of this; for I recollected turning up first one side and then the other, in search of the cleanest spot. Had the skull been then there, of course I could not have failed to notice it. Here was indeed a mystery which I felt it impossible to explain; but, even at that early moment, there it seemed to glimmer, faintly, within the most remote and secret chambers of my intellect, a glow-worm-like conception of that truth which last night's adventure brought to so magnificent a demonstration. I arose at once, and putting the parchment securely away, dismissed all farther reflection until I should be alone.

"When you had gone, and when Jupiter was fast asleep, I betook myself to a more methodical investigation of the affair. In the first place I considered the manner in which the parchment had come into my possession. The spot where we discovered the scarabaeus was on the coast of the main land, about a mile eastward of the island, and but a short distance above high water mark. Upon my taking hold of it, it gave me a sharp bite, which caused me to let it drop. Jupiter, with his accustomed caution, before seizing the insect, which had flown towards him, looked about him for a leaf, or something of that nature, by which to take hold of it.

It was at this moment that his eyes, and mine also, fell upon the scrap of parchment, which I then supposed to be paper. It was lying half buried in the sand, a corner sticking up. Near the spot where we found it, I observed the remnants of the hull of what appeared to have been a ship's long boat. The wreck seemed to have been there for a very great while; for the resemblance to boat timbers could scarcely be traced.

"Well, Jupiter picked up the parchment, wrapped the beetle in it, and gave it to me. Soon afterwards we turned to go home, and on the way met Lieutenant G--. I showed him the insect, and he begged me to let him take it to the fort. On my consenting, he thrust it forthwith into his waistcoat pocket, without the parchment in which it had been wrapped, and which I had continued to hold in my hand during his inspection. Perhaps he dreaded my changing my mind, and thought it best to make sure of the prize at once --you know how enthusiastic he is on all subjects connected with Natural History. At the same time without being conscious of it, I must have deposited the parchment in my own pocket.

"You remember that when I went to the table, for the purpose of making a sketch of the beetle, I found no paper where it was usually kept. I looked in the drawer, and found none there. I searched my pockets, hoping to find an old letter --and then my hand fell upon the parchment. I thus detail the precise mode in which it came into my possession; for the circumstances impressed me with peculiar force.

"No doubt you will think me fanciful --but I had already established a kind of connexion. I had put together two links of a great chain. There was a boat lying on a sea-coast, and not far from the boat was a parchment --not a paper --with a skull depicted on it. You will, of course, ask 'where is the connexion?' I reply that the skull, or death's-head, is the well-known emblem of the pirate. The flag of the death's-head is hoisted in all engagements.

"I have said that the scrap was parchment, and not paper. Parchment is durable --almost imperishable. Matters of little moment are rarely consigned to parchment; since, for the mere ordinary purposes of drawing or writing, it is not nearly so well adapted as paper. This reflection suggested some meaning -- some relevancy --in the death's-head. I did not fail to observe, also, the form of the parchment. Although one of its corners had been, by some accident, destroyed, it could be seen that the original form was oblong. It was just such a slip, indeed, as might have been chosen for a memorandum --for a record of something to be long remembered and carefully preserved."

"But," I interposed, "you say that the skull was not upon the parchment when you made the drawing of the beetle. How then do you trace any connexion between the boat and the skull --since this latter, according to your own admission, must have been designed (God only knows how or by whom) at some period subsequent to your sketching the scarabaeus?"

"Ah, hereupon turns the whole mystery; although the secret, at this point, I had comparatively little difficulty in solving. My steps were sure, and could afford but a single result. I reasoned, for example, thus: When I drew the scarabaeus, there was no skull apparent on the parchment. When I had completed the drawing, I gave it to you, and observed you narrowly until you returned it. You, therefore, did not design the skull, and no one else was present to do it. Then it was not done by human agency. And nevertheless it was done.

"At this stage of my reflections I endeavored to remember, and did remember, with entire distinctness, every incident which occurred about the period in question. The weather was chilly (oh rare and happy accident!), and a fire was blazing on the hearth. I was heated with exercise and sat near the table. You, however, had drawn a chair close to the chimney. Just as I placed the parchment in your hand, and as you were in the act of inspecting it, Wolf, the Newfoundland, entered, and leaped upon your shoulders. With your left hand you caressed him and kept him off, while your right, holding the parchment, was permitted to fall listlessly between your knees, and in close proximity to the fire. At one moment I thought the blaze had caught it, and was about to caution you, but, before I could speak, you had withdrawn it, and were engaged in its examination. When I considered all these particulars, I doubted not for a moment that heat had been the agent in bringing to light, on the parchment, the skull which I saw designed on it. You are well aware that chemical preparations exist, and have existed time out of mind, by means of which it is possible to write on either paper or vellum, so that the characters shall become visible only when subjected to the action of fire. Zaire, digested in aqua regia, and diluted with four times its weight of water, is sometimes employed; a green tint results. The regulus of cobalt, dissolved in spirit of nitre, gives a red. These colors disappear at longer or shorter intervals after the material written on cools, but again become apparent upon the re-application of heat.

"I now scrutinized the death's-head with care. Its outer edges --the edges of the drawing nearest the edge of the vellum --were far more distinct than the others. It was clear that the action of the caloric had been imperfect or unequal. I immediately kindled a fire, and subjected every portion of the parchment to a glowing heat. At first, the only effect was the strengthening of the faint lines in the skull; but, on persevering in the experiment, there became visible, at the corner of the slip, diagonally opposite to the spot in which the death's-head was delineated, the figure of what I at first supposed to be a goat. A closer scrutiny, however, satisfied me that it was intended for a kid."

225

"Ha! ha!" said I, "to be sure I have no right to laugh at you --a million and a half of money is too serious a matter for mirth --but you are not about to establish a third link in your chain --you will not find any especial connexion between your pirates and goat -- pirates, you know, have nothing to do with goats; they appertain to the farming interest."

"But I have just said that the figure was not that of a goat."

"Well, a kid then --pretty much the same thing."

"Pretty much, but not altogether," said Legrand. "You may have heard of one Captain Kidd. I at once looked on the figure of the animal as a kind of punning or hieroglyphical signature. I say signature; because its position on the vellum suggested this idea. The death's-head at the corner diagonally opposite, had, in the same manner, the air of a stamp, or seal. But I was sorely put out by the absence of all else --of the body to my imagined instrument --of the text for my context."

"I presume you expected to find a letter between the stamp and the signature."

"Something of that kind. The fact is, I felt irresistibly impressed with a presentiment of some vast good fortune impending. I can scarcely say why. Perhaps, after all, it was rather a desire than an actual belief; -- but do you know that Jupiter's silly words, about the bug being of solid gold, had a remarkable effect on my fancy? And then the series of accidents and coincidences --these were so very extraordinary. Do you observe how mere an accident it was that these events should have occurred on the sole day of all the year in which it has been, or may be, sufficiently cool for fire, and that without the fire, or without the intervention of the dog at the precise moment in which he appeared, I should never have become aware of the death's-head, and so never the possessor of the treasure?"

"But proceed --I am all impatience."

"Well; you have heard, of course, the many stories current --the thousand vague rumors afloat about money buried, somewhere on the Atlantic coast, by Kidd and his associates. These rumors must have had some foundation in fact. And that the rumors have existed so long and so continuously could have resulted, it appeared to me, only from the circumstance of the buried treasure still remaining entombed. Had Kidd concealed his plunder for a time, and afterwards reclaimed it, the rumors would scarcely have reached us in their present unvarying form. You will observe that the stories told are all about money-seekers, not about money-finders. Had the pirate recovered his money, there the affair would have dropped. It seemed to me that some accident -- say the loss of a memorandum indicating its locality --had deprived him of the means of recovering it, and that this accident had become known to is followers, who otherwise might never have heard that treasure had been concealed at all, and who, busying themselves in vain, because unguided attempts, to regain it, had given first birth, and then universal currency, to the reports which are now so common. Have you ever heard of any important treasure being unearthed along the coast?"

"Never."

"But that Kidd's accumulations were immense, is well known. I took it for granted, therefore, that the earth still held them; and you will scarcely be surprised when I tell you that I felt a hope, nearly amounting to certainty, that the parchment so strangely found, involved a lost record of the place of deposit."

"But how did you proceed?"

"I held the vellum again to the fire, after increasing the heat; but nothing appeared. I now thought it possible that the coating of dirt might have something to do with the failure; so I carefully rinsed the parchment by pouring warm water over it, and, having done this, I placed it in a tin pan, with the skull downwards, and put the pan upon a furnace of lighted charcoal. In a few minutes, the pan having become thoroughly heated, I removed the slip, and, to my inexpressible joy, found it spotted, in several places, with what appeared to be figures arranged in lines. Again I placed it in the pan, and suffered it to

228

remain another minute. On taking it off, the whole was just as you see it now."

Here Legrand, having re-heated the parchment, submitted It my inspection. The following characters were rudely traced, in a red tint, between the death's-head and the goat:

```
53++!305))6*;4826)4+.)4+);806*;48!8`60))85;
]8*:+*8!83(88)5*!;

46(;88*96*?;8)*+(;485);5*!2:*+(;4956*2(5*-
4)8`8*; 4069285);)6

!8)4++;1(+9;48081;8:8+1;48!85;4)485!528806*
81(+9;48;(88;4(+?3
   4;48)4+;161;:188;+?;
```

"But," said I, returning him the slip, "I am as much in the dark as ever. Were all the jewels of Golconda awaiting me on my solution of this enigma, I am quite sure that I should be unable to earn them."

; "And yet," said Legrand, "the solution is by no means so difficult as you might be led to imagine from the first hasty inspection of the characters. These characters, as any one might readily guess, form a cipher --that is to say, they convey a meaning; but then, from what is known of Kidd, I could not suppose him capable of constructing any of the more abstruse cryptographs. I made up my mind, at once, that this was of a simple species --such, however, as

229

would appear, to the crude intellect of the sailor, absolutely insoluble without the key."

"And you really solved it?"

"Readily; I have solved others of an abstruseness ten thousand times greater. Circumstances, and a certain bias of mind, have led me to take interest in such riddles, and it may well be doubted whether human ingenuity can construct an enigma of the kind which human ingenuity may not, by proper application, resolve. In fact, having once established connected and legible characters, I scarcely gave a thought to the mere difficulty of developing their import.

"In the present case --indeed in all cases of secret writing --the first question regards the language of the cipher; for the principles of solution, so far, especially, as the more simple ciphers are concerned, depend on, and are varied by, the genius of the particular idiom. In general, there is no alternative but experiment (directed by probabilities) of every tongue known to him who attempts the solution, until the true one be attained. But, with the cipher now before us, all difficulty is removed by the signature. The pun on the word 'Kidd' is appreciable in no other language than the English. But for this consideration I should have begun my attempts with the Spanish and French, as the tongues in which a secret of this kind would most naturally have been written by a pirate of the Spanish main. As it was, I assumed the cryptograph to be English.

"You observe there are no divisions between the words. Had there been divisions, the task would have been comparatively easy. In such case I should have commenced with a collation and analysis of the shorter words, and, had a word of a single letter occurred, as is most likely, (a or I, for example,) I should have considered the solution as assured. But, there being no division, my first step was to ascertain the predominant letters, as well as the least frequent. Counting all, I constructed a table, thus:

```
Of the character 8 there are 33.
                  ;       "    26.
                  4       "    19.
              + )         "    16.
                  *       "    13.
                  5       "    12.
                  6       "    11.
              ! 1         "     8.
                  0       "     6.
              9 2         "     5.
              : 3         "     4.
                  ?       "     3.
                  `       "     2.
              - .         "     1.
```

"Now, in English, the letter which most frequently occurs is e. Afterwards, the succession runs thus: *a o i d h n r s t u y c f g l m w b k p q x z*. E however predominates so remarkably that an individual sentence of any length is rarely seen, in which it is not the prevailing character.

; "Here, then, we have, in the very beginning, the groundwork for something more than a mere guess. The general use which may be made of the table is obvious --but, in this particular cipher, we shall only very partially require its aid. As our predominant character is 8, we will commence by assuming it as the e of the natural alphabet. To verify the supposition, let us observe if the 8 be seen often in couples --for e is doubled with great frequency in English --in such words, for example, as 'meet,' 'fleet,' 'speed, 'seen,' 'been,' 'agree,' &c. In the present instance we see it doubled less than five times, although the cryptograph is brief.

"Let us assume 8, then, as e. Now, of all words in the language, 'the' is the most usual; let us see, therefore, whether they are not repetitions of any three characters in the same order of collocation, the last of them being 8. If we discover repetitions of such letters, so arranged, they will most probably represent the word 'the.' On inspection, we find no less than seven such arrangements, the characters being ;48. We may, therefore, assume that the semicolon represents t, that 4 represents h, and that 8 represents e --the last being now well confirmed. Thus a great step has been taken.

"But, having established a single word, we are enabled to establish a vastly important point; that is to say, several commencements and terminations of other words. Let us refer, for example, to the last instance but one, in which the combination ;48 occurs

--not far from the end of the cipher. We know that the semicolon immediately ensuing is the commencement of a word, and, of the six characters succeeding this 'the,' we are cognizant of no less than five. Let us set these characters down, thus, by the letters we know them to represent, leaving a space for the unknown--

t eeth.

; "Here we are enabled, at once, to discard the 'th,' as forming no portion of the word commencing with the first t; since, by experiment of the entire alphabet for a letter adapted to the vacancy we perceive that no word can be formed of which this th can be a part. We are thus narrowed into

t ee,

and, going through the alphabet, if necessary, as before, we arrive at the word 'tree,' as the sole possible reading. We thus gain another letter, r, represented by (, with the words 'the tree' in juxtaposition.

; "Looking beyond these words, for a short distance, we again see the combination ;48, and employ it by way of termination to what immediately precedes. We have thus this arrangement:

the tree ;4(+?34 the,

or substituting the natural letters, where known, it reads thus:

the tree thr+?3h the.

; "Now, if, in place of the unknown characters, we leave blank spaces, or substitute dots, we read thus:

the tree thr...h the,

when the word 'through' makes itself evident at once. But this discovery gives us three new letters, o, u and g, represented by + ? and 3.

; "Looking now, narrowly, through the cipher for combinations of known characters, we find, not very far from the beginning, this arrangement,

83(88, or egree,

which, plainly, is the conclusion of the word 'degree,' and gives us another letter, d, represented by !.

; "Four letters beyond the word 'degree,' we perceive the combination

;46(;88*.

; "Translating the known characters, and representing the unknown by dots, as before, we read thus:

th.rtee.

an arrangement immediately suggestive of the word 'thirteen,' and again furnishing us with two new characters, i and n, represented by 6 and *.

; "Referring, now, to the beginning of the cryptograph, we find the combination,

53++!.

; "Translating, as before, we obtain

.good,

which assures us that the first letter is A, and that the first two words are 'A good.'

; "To avoid confusion, it is now time that we arrange our key, as far as discovered, in a tabular form. It will stand thus:

```
5 represents a
!      "       d
8      "       e
3      "       g
4      "       h
6      "       i
*      "       n
+      "       o
(      "       r
;      "       t
```

"We have, therefore, no less than ten of the most important letters represented, and it will be unnecessary to proceed with the details of the solution. I have said enough to convince you that ciphers of this nature are readily soluble, and to give you some insight into the rationale of their development. But be assured that the specimen before us appertains to the very simplest species of cryptograph. It now only remains to give you the full translation of the characters upon the parchment, as unriddled. Here it is:

; 'A good glass in the bishop's hostel in the devil's seat twenty-one degrees and thirteen minutes northeast and by north main branch seventh limb east side shoot from the left eye of the death's-head a bee line from the tree through the shot fifty feet out.'"

; "But," said I, "the enigma seems still in as bad a condition as ever. How is it possible to extort a meaning from all this jargon about 'devil's seats,' 'death's-heads,' and 'bishop's hostel'?"

"I confess," replied Legrand, "that the matter still wears a serious aspect, when regarded with a casual glance. My first endeavor was to divide the sentence into the natural division intended by the cryptographist."

"You mean, to punctuate it?"

"Something of that kind."

"But how was it possible to effect this?"

"I reflected that it had been a point with the writer to run his words together without division, so as to increase the difficulty of solution. Now, a not overacute man, in pursuing such an object, would be nearly certain to overdo the matter. When, in the course of his composition, he arrived at a break in his subject which would naturally require a pause, or a point, he would be exceedingly apt to run his characters, at this place, more than usually close together. If you will observe the MS., in the present instance, you will easily detect five such cases of unusual crowding. Acting on this hint, I made the division thus:

; 'A good glass in the bishop's hostel in the devil's -- twenty-one degrees and thirteen minutes --northeast and by north --main branch seventh limb east side -- shoot from the left eye of the death's-head --a bee-line from the tree through the shot fifty feet out.'"

; "Even this division," said I, "leaves me still in the dark."

"It left me also in the dark," replied Legrand, "for a few days; during which I made diligent inquiry, in the neighborhood of Sullivan's Island, for any building which went by the name of the 'Bishop's Hotel'; for, of course, I dropped the obsolete word 'hostel.' Gaining no information on the subject, I was on the point of extending my sphere of search, and proceeding in a more systematic manner, when, one morning, it entered into my head, quite suddenly, that this 'Bishop's Hostel' might have some reference to an old family, of the name of Bessop, which, time out of mind, had held possession of an ancient manor-house, about four miles to the northward of the Island. I accordingly went over to the plantation, and reinstituted my inquiries among the older negroes of the place. At length one of the most aged of the women said that she had heard of such a place as Bessop's Castle, and thought that she could guide me to it, but that it was not a castle, nor a tavern, but a high rock.

"I offered to pay her well for her trouble, and, after some demur, she consented to accompany me to the spot. We found it without much difficulty, when, dismissing her, I proceeded to examine the place. The 'castle' consisted of an irregular assemblage of cliffs and rocks --one of the latter being quite remarkable for its height as well as for its insulated and artificial appearance. I clambered to its apex, and then felt much at a loss as to what should be next done.

"While I was busied in reflection, my eyes fell upon a narrow ledge in the eastern face of the rock, perhaps a yard below the summit on which I stood. This ledge projected about eighteen inches, and was not more than a foot wide, while a niche in the cliff just above it, gave it a rude resemblance to one of the hollow-backed chairs used by our ancestors. I made no doubt that here was the 'devil's-seat' alluded to in the MS., and now I seemed to grasp the full secret of the riddle.

"The 'good glass,' I knew, could have reference to nothing but a telescope; for the word 'glass' is rarely employed in any other sense by seamen. Now here, I at once saw, was a telescope to be used, and a definite point of view, admitting no variation, from which to use it. Nor did I hesitate to believe that the phrases, 'twenty-one degrees and thirteen minutes,' and northeast and by north,' were intended as directions for the levelling of the glass. Greatly excited by these discoveries, I hurried home, procured a telescope, and returned to the rock.

"I let myself down to the ledge, and found that it was impossible to retain a seat on it unless in one particular position. This fact confirmed my preconceived idea. I proceeded to use the glass. Of course, the 'twenty-one degrees and thirteen minutes' could allude to nothing but elevation above the visible horizon, since the horizontal direction was clearly indicated by the words, 'northeast and by north.' This latter direction I at once established by means of a pocket-compass; then, pointing the glass as nearly at an angle of twenty-one degrees of elevation as I could do it by guess, I moved it cautiously up or down, until my attention was arrested by a circular rift or opening in the foliage of a large tree that overtopped its fellows in the distance. In the centre of this rift I perceived a white spot, but could not, at first, distinguish what it was. Adjusting the focus of the telescope, I again looked, and now made it out to be a human skull.

"On this discovery I was so sanguine as to consider the enigma solved; for the phrase 'main branch, seventh limb, east side,' could refer only to the position of the skull on the tree, while shoot from the left eye of the death's-head' admitted, also, of but one interpretation, in regard to a search for buried treasure. I perceived that the design was to drop a bullet from the left eye of the skull, and that a bee-line, or, in other words, a straight line, drawn from the nearest point of the trunk through 'the shot,' (or the spot where the bullet fell,) and thence extended to a distance of fifty feet, would indicate a definite point --and beneath this point I thought it at least possible that a deposit of value lay concealed."

"All this," I said, "is exceedingly clear, and, although ingenious, still simple and explicit. When you left the Bishop's Hotel, what then?"

"Why, having carefully taken the bearings of the tree, I turned homewards. The instant that I left 'the devil's seat,' however, the circular rift vanished; nor could I get a glimpse of it afterwards, turn as I would. What seems to me the chief ingenuity in this whole business, is the fact (for repeated experiment has convinced me it is a fact) that the circular opening in question is visible from no other attainable point of view than that afforded by the narrow ledge on the face of the rock.

"In this expedition to the 'Bishop's Hotel' I had been attended by Jupiter, who had, no doubt, observed, for some weeks past, the abstraction of my demeanor, and took especial care not to leave me alone. But, on the next day, getting up very early, I contrived to give him the slip, and went into the hills in search of the tree. After much toil I found it. When I came home at night my valet proposed to give me a flogging. With the rest of the adventure I believe you are as well acquainted as myself."

"I suppose," said I, "you missed the spot, in the first attempt at digging through Jupiter's stupidity in letting the bug fall through the right instead of the left of the skull."

"Precisely. This mistake made a difference of about two inches and a half in the 'shot' --that is to say, in the position of the peg nearest the tree; and had the treasure been beneath the 'shot,' the error would have been of little moment; but the 'shot,' together with the nearest point of the tree, were merely two points for the establishment of a line of direction; of course the error, however trivial in the beginning, increased as we proceeded with the line, and by the time we had gone fifty feet, threw us quite off the scent. But for my deep-seated convictions that treasure was here somewhere actually buried, we might have had all our labor in vain."

"I presume the fancy of the skull, of letting fall a bullet through the skull's eye --was suggested to Kidd by the piratical flag. No doubt he felt a kind of poetical consistency in recovering his money through this ominous insignium."

"Perhaps so; still I cannot help thinking that common-sense had quite as much to do with the matter as poetical consistency. To be visible from the devil's-seat, it was necessary that the object, if small, should be white; and there is nothing like your human skull for retaining and even increasing its whiteness under exposure to all vicissitudes of weather."

"But your grandiloquence, and your conduct in swinging the beetle --how excessively odd! I was sure you were mad. And why did you insist on letting fall the bug, instead of a bullet, from the skull?"

"Why, to be frank, I felt somewhat annoyed by your evident suspicions touching my sanity, and so resolved to punish you quietly, in my own way, by a little bit of sober mystification. For this reason I swung the beetle, and for this reason I let it fall from the tree. An observation of yours about its great weight suggested the latter idea."

"Yes, I perceive; and now there is only one point which puzzles me. What are we to make of the skeletons found in the hole?"

"That is a question I am no more able to answer than yourself. There seems, however, only one plausible way of accounting for them --and yet it is dreadful to believe in such atrocity as my suggestion would imply. It is clear that Kidd --if Kidd indeed secreted this treasure, which I doubt not --it is clear that he must have had assistance in the labor. But, the worst of this labor concluded, he may have thought it expedient to remove all participants in his secret. Perhaps a couple of blows with a mattock were sufficient, while his coadjutors were busy in the pit; perhaps it required a dozen --who shall tell?"

Other books from **MAGIC LAMP PRESS**:

By **EDWIN H. SINCLAIR, Jr.**

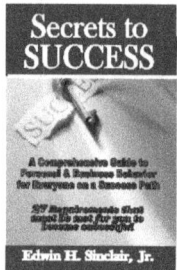 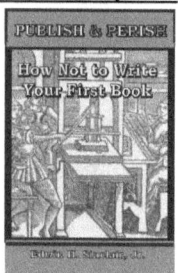 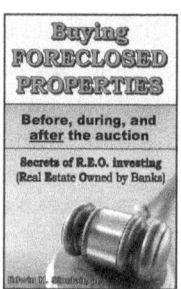

SECRETS TO PERSONAL SUCCESS
PUBLISH & PERISH
BUYING FORECLOSED PROPERTIES

By **Dr. NICK SHOVEEN, Ph.D.**

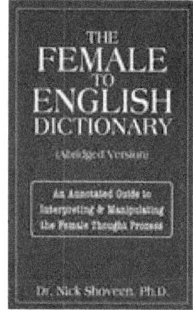 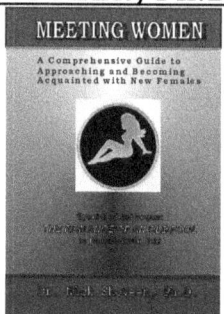 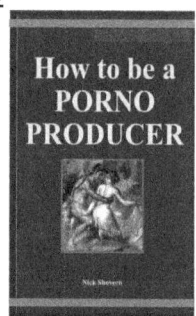

The FEMALE-to-ENGLISH DICTIONARY
A GUIDE to MEETING WOMEN
HOW TO BE A PORNO PRODUCER

By **BARRY NEAL**

Get Started & Manage Your Comedy Career

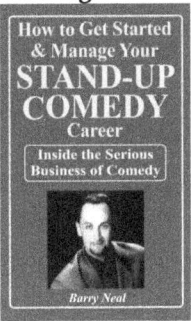

Magic Lamp Press also offers several classic books that are now available for your pleasure.

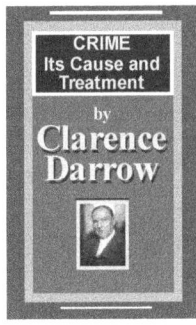

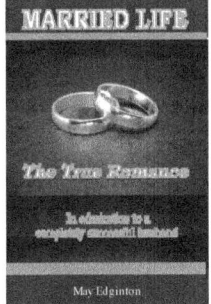

Full details for all of these books, as well as the entire 10-book set of Peter Sharp Legal Mysteries are at:
www.magiclampdigital.com

www.ingramcontent.com/pod-product-compliance
Lightning Source LLC
Chambersburg PA
CBHW070817180626
46818CB00001B/302